TRUTH
BODY SOLUTIONS

ALSO BY FRANK SEPE

FRANK SEPE'S ABS-OLUTELY PERFECT PLAN FOR A FLATTER STOMACH:
The <u>Only</u> Abs Book You'll Ever Need!

THE TRUTH: The <u>Only</u> Fitness Book You'll Ever Need

HAY HOUSE TITLES OF RELATED INTEREST

BODYCHANGE™: The 21-Day Fitness Program
for Changing Your Body . . . and Changing Your Life!,
by Montel Williams and Wini Linguvic

8 MINUTES IN THE MORNING®TO A FLAT BELLY KIT:
Lose Up to 6 Inches in Less Than 4 Weeks—Guaranteed!,
by Jorge Cruise

THE NATIONAL BODY CHALLENGE™ SUCCESS
PROGRAM FOR THE WHOLE FAMILY,
by Pamela Peeke, M.D., M.P.H., F.A.C.P.

SHAPE® MAGAZINE'S ULTIMATE BODY BOOK:
4 Weeks to Your Best Abs, Butt, Thighs, and More!,
by Linda Shelton, with Angela Hynes

TRANSFORMATION: How to Change EVERYTHING,
by Bill Phillips (available October 2006)

ULTIMATE PILATES, by Dreas Reyneke

WHAT ARE YOU REALLY EATING?:
How to Become Label Savvy, by Amanda Ursell

YOGA PURE AND SIMPLE, by Kisen

All of the above are available at your local
bookstore, or may be ordered by visiting:

Hay House USA: **www.hayhouse.com**®
Hay House Australia: **www.hayhouse.com.au**
Hay House UK: **www.hayhouse.co.uk**
Hay House South Africa: **orders@psdprom.co.za**
Hay House India: **www.hayhouseindia.co.in**

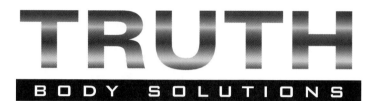

TRUTH
BODY SOLUTIONS

Truthful Nutritional
Strategies for a
Better Body and
a Better Life

FRANK SEPE

HAY HOUSE, INC.
Carlsbad, California
London • Sydney • Johannesburg
Vancouver • Hong Kong • Mumbai

Library of Congress Cataloging-in-Publication Data

Sepe, Frank.
  Truth body solutions: truthful nutritional strategies for a better body and a
better life / Frank Sepe.
      p. cm.
  ISBN-13: 978-1-4019-1048-8 (tradepaper)
  ISBN-10: 1-4019-1048-3 (tradepaper)
  1. Reducing diets. 2. Reducing exercises. 3. Weight loss. 4. Weight gain. 5.
Bodybuilding. I. Title.

  RM222.2.S43 2006
  613.7'12--dc22
                                  2005032103

                    ISBN 13: 978-1-4019-1048-8
                    ISBN 10: 1-4019-1048-3

                   09 08 07 06   4 3 2 1
                        1st printing, May 2006

                Printed in the United States of America

I dedicate this book to Rocky Sepe—
the best training partner I've ever had.
Rest in peace, buddy.
You will never be forgotten.

CONTENTS

Introduction...ix

PART I: THE **TRUTH** ABOUT WEIGHT LOSS

Introduction to Part I.. 3
Chapter 1:   The TRUTH Will Set You Free from Diets 5
Chapter 2:   And Now a Word from Your Metabolism 13
Chapter 3:   The TRUTH Eating Plan..................................... 19
Chapter 4:   Weight-Loss Q & A.. 43

PART II: THE **TRUTH** ABOUT WEIGHT GAIN

Introduction to Part II..51
Chapter 5:   What Is Skinny, Anyway? 53
Chapter 6:   The Dangers of Being Underweight................. 57
Chapter 7:   No Loss—All Gain... 63
Chapter 8:   The TRUTH Weight-Gain Plan 67
Chapter 9:   Weight-Gain Q & A 81

PART III: THE **TRUTH** ABOUT MUSCLE BUILDING

Introduction to Part III..91
Chapter 10:   Muscle-Building 101.. 93
Chapter 11:   How Bodybuilders "Muscle Up" 101
Chapter 12:   Sports-Nutrition Products 105
Chapter 13:   The TRUTH Muscle-Building Plan.................... 111
Chapter 14:   Muscle-Building Q & A.................................... 127

APPENDIX

Bonus Chapter: Training 101.. 137
A Final Word on Cardio and Calorie Burning 141
The MET-Rx/Frank Sepe DVD.. 151
My Personal Plan 155
The TRUTH Master Food List.. 157
About the Author 163

INTRODUCTION

Can you handle The TRUTH?

That's not just a take on the line Jack Nicholson used on Tom Cruise at the end of one of my favorite courtroom thrillers, *A Few Good Men*—it's also what I ask my clients, who come to me for my very unique personal-training program, which I happen to call "The TRUTH." (I'll tell you what the letters stand for in just a minute.)

Right now I'd like to start by putting honesty on hold for a few minutes and focus instead on the lies we all tell ourselves when it comes to fitness. Never was this more apparent to me than on a recent Sunday when I went to my local bookstore outside of New York City.

A couple I'll call Joe and Jane Smith rushed through the revolving door with me. They were your typical suburbanites in their late 30s, talking loudly about their joint mission.

"We need to go on a serious diet, Joe," Jane said. "I just can't stand being this fat anymore."

"Honey, you're not fat," Joe replied without skipping a beat. Secretly, I give this guy his props, because every husband in America knows that this line should basically be part of the new marriage vows: "I promise to love, honor, respect you, and tell you on a daily basis that your butt looks really great in those jeans."

Back to the Smiths. They carefully made sure that the store was devoid of any neighbors, friends, or anyone else who's ever known them. When the coast was clear, they entered the "Health and Fitness" section of the store. Going there is like an alcoholic going to his first AA meeting: It's the first step in admitting that a major life change is needed. I also really feel that everyone should be applauded for having this type of courage.

On a stealth mission to see what they'd do in the name of fitness, I followed Joe and Jane and noticed that they looked completely befuddled. In front of them was a virtual wall of information, and they began to give their fingers a good workout by letting them do the walking through the large collection of titles. Jane didn't believe that she could lose 50 pounds in two minutes a day, while Joe didn't think that he could eat raw asparagus for the rest of his life in order to get rid of the tire around his stomach—he's just not a vegetable person. And both of them agreed that belly dancing their way to new bodies just wasn't their style.

Finding a few books that they could relate to a little more, Joe and Jane took them to the little café in the bookstore, where they planned to decide on the diet plan that would help them become hot and buff and would extend their lives . . . and that's when it happened.

"Honey, I'll go get us a couple of muffins and Frappuccinos while you look at the books," Joe said, getting $20 out of his wallet. (Why is it that all the food that's bad for you is always expensive?)

"No whipped cream," Jane said, feeling better about her coffee treat because she saved about 30 calories from one hit of Reddi-wip. It's like ordering a Diet Coke with your triple-hot-fudge sundae!

Balancing about 2,000 calories worth of snacks in his hand, Joe eventually joined Jane at their little table. "Our diet starts tomorrow!" she vowed, as her husband put extra sugar in his coffee and took a giant bite out of his muffin.

Now, let's go back to The **TRUTH** of the matter.

My guess is that Jane and Joe have messed with another famous movie line. For them, tomorrow's another day . . . to start their diet-and-exercise plan.

Unfortunately, tomorrow never really comes, and in its place are about ten new pounds every six months, a bunch of bumpy cellulite patches, and this nagging feeling that they're becoming tired and sluggish for no real reason.

Welcome to the standard "diet plan" of most Americans.

Well, tomorrow finally *has* come for you, in the form of this book. If you agree not to go back to your fitness yesterdays, I'll bet that you'll have the type of body you've always wanted. And I'm sorry to report that the side effects will only be more energy, better sleep at night, and a feeling of vigor that you probably haven't experienced in years.

Repeat after me: "No, I'm not supposed to be this tired and sluggish." It's time to get rid of those feelings forever, while also achieving the type of body that you never even thought was possible.

My name is Frank Sepe, and I'll promise you two things right now: First, I'll always be straight up with you when it comes to your diet-and-exercise program; and second, if you stick with me, you'll never be in that confusing section of the bookstore again.

I've said it before, but it bears repeating: My fitness program is the last one you'll ever need. Can you handle *that* TRUTH? I thought you could.

When I sat down to write this book, the first words that went through my mind were the obvious: *Great, just what the world needs—another book about eating right and exercising.* But this actually is exactly what the world needs. We must have one last definitive book to start on a path to health and finally achieve the body of our dreams.

And for those of you who purchased my other two books, let me say thanks for your trust. I know from the thousands of letters I've received that the plan is working for women and men from all different walks of life. Young and old, single and married, moms and dads, and kids and teenagers all know that there's only one TRUTH when it comes to diet and exercise. And that is:

T: The Time is Now!
You have to decide that there's no time like the present to start on this program.

R: Reality Check
I'll help clear up any misconceptions that might have stopped you from seeing the results you want from a health-and-fitness regimen.

U: Unleash Your Mental Power
A proper program goes much deeper than just getting your body in shape—it begins with your mind and making a commitment to a new lifestyle.

T: Train, Train, Train
This one's pretty self-explanatory!

H: Healthy Eating
The final component to The TRUTH is a meal plan in which you can eat healthy foods that work hand-in-hand with your training program to help you look and feel fantastic.

But now it's time to amp it up a little bit and fine-tune your program for maximum results. This new book is divided into three parts: weight loss, weight gain, and muscle building. You'll need to choose which of the first two sections apply to your individual needs: Do you want to take off a few pounds or bulk up a bit? For those who want to lose weight, I'll discuss diet and nutritional plans, metabolism, and roadblocks to weight loss, and I'll also offer solid and healthy advice that's easy, safe, and effective. My objective is to give you truthful nutritional strategies that will help you lose the weight permanently.

If you're one of those people who longs to gain a few pounds, don't despair! We'll take a different approach to this challenge: I'll teach you how to put on some bulk without jeopardizing your health. I want to help you permanently gain the weight you want while building muscle at the same time.

In both cases, I'll explain what to eat and drink and when to use specific nutritional products that may help with your progress. We'll come back together for the third part of the book, which will be muscle building. Remember that this doesn't mean getting big and burly—it's about *sculpting* muscles to burn fat and have a sleeker body. This segment isn't for bodybuilders, but simply for those who want a more defined physique.

Each section will be filled with information-packed sidebars that will help keep you on your program, along with an actual eating and/or muscle-building plan. And a chapter at the end of each part will contain several of the most common questions on what we've just discussed.

The book also features a special DVD sponsored by MET-Rx, in which I take you through some of my very favorite beginning- and intermediate-workout routines. This will be like making an appointment with me for a personal session, since I've put together a simple routine that can be accomplished in your home with simple weights and a workout bench. Fitness doesn't have to be complicated or costly—my goal is to get you moving on a regular basis. Once you begin to see the results, then I know that you'll want to continue on in a commercial gym.

Our goal will be to build muscle, which will shape your body and also keep the weight off . . . talk about a win-win situation!

FOR THOSE OF YOU WHO DON'T KNOW ME, allow me to give you a quick introduction. I was a scrawny kid from New York whose father had a glorious workout room in our basement. Little kids like me were told to keep out, but I wasn't very good at listening to the rules. When I was about 13, I started sneaking down there and working the weights, not exactly knowing what I was doing, but enjoying putting a little meat on my frame.

When my father figured out what was going on, he wasn't mad, but he did sit me down and begin to teach me the principles of weight lifting. Fascinated by muscle building and health, I spent the next decade studying the human form, discovering what works to shape a body, and then applying it to clients and myself. I've been a bodybuilder and a spokesperson for MET-Rx, plus you might have seen my smiling face on ESPN2's show *Cold Pizza.* As a trainer, I've worked with the rich and famous, along with just regular men and women, because we all have the same goals: We want to look and feel great, and no amount of money can beat that feeling.

I've been on the fitness front line for the last 15 years, and I want to show you what I've learned by training thousands of people with vastly different body types. When I meet my clients, they seem to have one thing in common: They're confused about where to turn in this gigantic fitness universe, which is now a multibillion-dollar industry.

Many of them have been on what I like to call the "diet-and-exercise treadmill"—they've tried all the programs out there for a short amount of time, seen few results, and quit in frustration. I've heard these words over and over again: "Frank, nothing seems to work for me."

Those days are over.

Remember that your body isn't like anyone else's in this entire world. One week you might seem to be making little progress, and then the next week it's like progress-palooza. Just go at your own pace, savor the moments, and enjoy your fitness victories.

NOW, LET'S GO BACK TO JOE AND JANE SMITH from the beginning of this chapter. After their muffins and designer coffees, they couldn't decide what fitness book to buy. Joe put down one of those 1,000-page books that he knew he'd never read and looked dejected. Jane glanced at another work with a half-nude model on the cover and knew that she'd never look that good in a million years. That's when they came up with another solution

"Do you want to just go out to lunch?" Joe asked his wife.

"Well, our diet hasn't started yet," Jane said in a wistful voice.

If only I could have reminded them that they've been saying the same thing for the last 30 weekends in a row. . . . If *you've* done the same thing, it's no big deal, but stop, take a breath, and make a vow to make today the beginning of the rest of your life. I promise that we'll have some fun along the way.

Just please skip the chocolate-chip muffin. Don't do it for me—do it for you.

□——□——□

PART I

THE **TRUTH**
ABOUT
WEIGHT
LOSS

I know what you're thinking, because in addition to being a top personal trainer, I'm also a mind reader. I can tell that you're internally fuming, *Oh, here we go again. This is just another thing that's going to pester me to eat the right way.*

It would be easy to just throw this book down and pick up a Twinkie—especially when you consider that your fellow Americans spend billions a year to take the newest pills, mix up the powers, chug the diet shakes, and eat two lettuces leaves for dinner, yet are fatter than ever.

Consider that as I write this book, 75 percent of adults in the United States are either trying to lose weight or keep themselves from gaining some extra pounds. Two out of three women and one out of two men are currently dieting. And sit down for this one: Some 95 percent of all dieters regain their lost weight. Isn't it time to stop the insanity?

In this section, I'll explain why your current program isn't working and why it can never help you shed pounds that will stay off for the rest of your life. After a little bit of necessary education about your body, I'll move on to give you a solid eating plan and then clear up any weight-loss questions that are on your mind. I'm not reading your mind again—I simply did an informal poll across America of what roadblocks most people come up against while trying to make their plan work.

Let's flip the page and start losing those pounds!

CHAPTER 1

THE **TRUTH** WILL SET YOU FREE FROM DIETS

It doesn't help to start any new plan unless you know what the motivation behind it is. So before you shed a single calorie, I'd like you to ask yourself one question: "Why do I want to lose weight?"

You may think that it's time to improve your looks, stun someone at a special occasion, improve your health, feel better in general, or change your life. Of course I can't promise you that weight loss will be the only catalyst in transforming your existence, but I've found that it's a good place to start. When you feel better about yourself for whatever reason, it trickles down to feeling good about your job, your family, your love life, and many other important aspects of the world.

If you're honest about why you want to lose weight, you can then focus on your true goals. It's fine if you say, "I want to shed some pounds so that my boyfriend will think I'm hot." That's certainly a good enough reason in my book. Other people might answer, "I want to get rid of some flab so that I can make it across a parking lot without feeling out of breath."

One woman told me that her doctor suggested that weight loss might help with her type 2 diabetes. (By the way, she shed 100 pounds and was actually taken off her medicine. She doesn't feel light-headed or tired anymore, and enjoys going off to the gym in the morning. A year ago, the same woman detested walking down her driveway.)

A guy once came to me with the idea of putting on a little muscle to counteract his middle-aged spread. I heard this one from a gal who was in her 50s, and it inspired me: "I want to go to my high school reunion and look so good that the boy who sat behind me in geometry class regrets not taking me to the prom." The same woman could still be saying, "I'm eating five doughnuts a day because some guy didn't take me to this dance 30 years ago," but she decided to take some action.

Like all my clients, if you've decided to lose weight, you have my respect—and my help. First, I'd like you to take out a piece of paper and write down three reasons why you want to lose weight. Keep this list in an area where you can look at it from time to time as you achieve your goals.

You're going to be so proud of yourself! I know that *I'm* already impressed with you.

A Body-Obsessed Society

Today we live in such a body-conscious society—after all, whom do you know who *isn't* obsessing about what the scale reads? And I guarantee that if you kept a log, at least ten times a day you'd note something that someone said on TV or in your life about weight control.

Think about it . . . you're eating a doughnut (the diet starts tomorrow) in your car on the way to work, and you hear a dozen commercials on the radio for weight-loss pills, metabolism boosters, low-carb hot fudge, and nonfat pork rolls. All of these announcers are spewing out sentences such as: "Lose weight fast! Lose weight easy! It only takes seconds a day! Delicious and low fat! Working out isn't necessary!"

Then you stop for coffee at a famous fast-food joint. You marvel at the new "alternative healthy menu" that promises only 30 grams of fat as opposed to the regular old 1,000 grams. You wonder, *Is 30 still too much? And will it make everything taste like cardboard?*

As you drive into your office, you notice super-slim, sexy models on billboards every two steps selling everything from cologne to fitness equipment to themselves. (And if you ride the bus, you can't even get on without seeing half a dozen health-club ads.) You might stop at your local newsstand for a magazine, but that can also be depressing because the latest celebrity du jour will be on the cover to promote how she or he lost weight or put on the muscle for a big-budget movie.

At the end of the day, you can finally relax in the comfort of your own home . . . or can you? You flip on the boob tube, only to hear about the latest gastric-bypass surgery. Even Larry King is talking about extreme makeovers and the plastic surgery of the stars. Jay Leno is listening to Teri Hatcher talk about how dancing around a strippers' pole made her thin, and you might try it, but the only pole in your neighborhood is attached to a street sign. Could you be arrested for dancing like Teri on the corner of your block?

Oprah Winfrey seems like a logical stop for some sanity, but then there's her ever-changing body. How *did* she lose that weight? Maybe you should follow her program, except you can't afford a trainer and a full-time cook. You flip the channel, and an infomercial promises that for $39.99 (in four convenient payments), they'll send you a book that will teach you to lose weight while you sleep.

As I said, we live in a very body-conscious society. I don't want you to diet to fit in with the pack, but instead, I'd like you to use this book to separate what's real about weight loss from what's just real nonsense.

BY THE NUMBERS:
WHY AMERICA NEEDS TO GO ON A DIET

- 400,000: The number of deaths relating to weight problems that occur per year.

- 39: The percentage of adults who aren't involved in any physical activity.

- 10 billion: The number of doughnuts consumed each year.

- 20.7: The pounds of candy ingested each year by the average American.

- 90: The percentage of children dining at fast-food restaurants each month.

- 1.2 billion: The pounds of potato chips eaten each year.

- $7 billion: The amount spent per year on chocolate.

- Fried chicken: The most commonly ordered restaurant meal.

- $60 billion: The amount spent on soft drinks in the year 2000.

- 15 billion: The number of gallons of soda consumed per year.

- $25 billion: The amount spent on beer per year.

- $50 billion: The number of dollars spent on weight-loss products.

WHY YOU NEED TO DROP THE POUNDS . . . STARTING TODAY

Losing weight and getting in shape isn't just about looking like Cameron Diaz. Of course, there are those who say, "Frank, I'm 25 pounds overweight and am happy with the way I look. I don't care what other people think—plus, people who live in the gym have no lives."

I've had many people also tell me, "I'd love to work out and stick to a diet plan, but with work and the kids, the best I can do is swing by McDonald's and then flop on the couch at night."

Well, let me be the first (and hopefully the last) one to convince you that there are very important reasons why you need to get a handle on your health right now. These reasons are actually *for* your children, and they're often more important than your nine-to-five job. Here's why you should lose the weight forever:

— **Your health.** It's a proven fact that overweight people tend to have health problems, including type 2 diabetes, high blood pressure, and heart and liver problems. As you age, it's not good for your frame or internal organs to be surrounded by masses of fat supported by muscles that are turning to jelly. The flip side is that losing weight through a nutritionally sound diet combined with exercise will actually make you healthier.

— **Increased energy.** With each pound of fat you lose, you'll feel a little bit better and have more energy. Think of it like carrying a heavy backpack full of bricks: Wouldn't you feel lighter and happier if you tossed out one brick, and then a second one? It's the same thing with your weight. Lose the pounds and you'll turn back the clock in terms of how much energy you have.

— **Longevity.** Your best chance of living longer is being in better condition. It makes sense that if you want to extend your life, then you need to shed the weight and keep it off.

— **Better sleep.** One of the best "side effects" of losing weight is that the fat won't compress your lungs at night when you sleep. Extremely overweight people actually have a condition known as *sleep apnea*—they don't get enough oxygen while they sleep, which leaves them feeling exhausted all the time. If *you* feel tired even after you've gotten eight hours of shut-eye, I promise that as you drop the pounds, you'll sleep better and wake up truly feeling refreshed and ready to go.

— **Higher self-esteem.** I don't want to sound shallow here, but it feels good to look great. I'm not promising that losing weight will change your life or get you that date or promotion, but it *will* lead to a jolt of self-esteem that will help you lead a better life. Plus, who doesn't want to go try on a smaller size when they walk into the Gap?

WHY DIETS DON'T WORK

Now that you're armed with your own personal motivation, it's time to come back together and talk about why diets don't work.

Let me explain the most important principle of weight loss: You need to consume fewer calories and increase physical activity to drop the pounds. If you do both of these things, then all the excess fat will simply fall off of you. This isn't some lofty promise, but a scientific, undisputable fact.

I'm not sure why people have made dieting so complicated, but maybe it's because we live in an age of wanting "the quick fix." People go on quickie diets like only eating apples for two days or restricting all carbs (more on that later) in an attempt to drop the pounds in the fastest way possible. These same people don't learn anything about nutrition, and also choose plans that are so rigid that they're doomed for failure.

You must *permanently* change your eating patterns in order to maintain a body that's healthy and in shape. I'm afraid that there aren't any shortcuts or magical pills or potions that will make this not be true. Again, those are just the facts of being a human being in a unique body.

You can't live by this phrase anymore: "I can just go on the latest fad diet and maintain a healthy, fit, trim body." Just say that once aloud—doesn't it seem ridiculous? Ask yourself why, then, do you try fad diet after fad diet when you know deep down that you'll never achieve your true body goals?

Okay, it's time to stop beating yourself up because those days are definitely over. Remember that despite what quick-fix diets promise, the only sensible way to lose the pounds and maintain a healthy weight for the rest of your life is to eat less and balance food intake with physical exercise.

Did you ever see a fat prehistoric person? That's because our early ancestors ate healthy meat and veggies and practically killed themselves trying to run from wild beasts in order to stay alive. They didn't have an easy life, but they achieved a healthy weight by eating less (food was hard to find), and balancing their food intake with regular physical exercise.

Oh, and moving your rolling office chair to the other side of the room with your toes does *not* constitute regular physical exercise.

FRANKLY SPEAKING: Did you know that at any minute of the day, two billion people are eating fast food? That's enough fried junk to make me want to scream! I call it the "oil slick around the world."

CHAPTER 2

AND NOW A WORD FROM YOUR METABOLISM

When I walk around the mall, I always do a little checkup of the people around me. You can try it, too. If you look around, I'll bet you notice that four out of five people are overweight and out of shape. And if you spoke to some of them, you might hear why weight has always been a stubborn problem, which would be a variation on what I often hear: "No matter what diet I try or how much working out I do, I can't lose weight because I've ruined my metabolism for life with all my crazy diets."

It's time to set the record straight concerning your metabolism. It's true that it does dictate how many calories you burn on the average day—however, it's not the true reason you're holding on to the weight. It's just the easiest thing to blame because you figure that there's really nothing you can do about it.

Many different factors determine what speed—high, medium, or low—your metabolism kicks into on an average day. First, you have to take heredity into consideration, which is the part you can't change. Okay, stop blaming your parents right now. Metabolism is also affected by age, level of activity, overall health, and the d-word *(diet)*, which I think we should all consider to be encouraging news.

You see, even if you think you have a so-so metabolism— an AMC Pacer of calorie burners, if you will—you can soup it up with the right diet and exercise. Let's say that you sit on the couch night after night with a family-sized bag of Cheetos in one hand and a beer in the other. When you go to unzip your jeans because they're feeling like someone put you into a straitjacket with two legs, please don't blame your metabolism, which doesn't know the phone number for the local take-out joint.

On the other hand, if you clean up your diet and start exercising, then your junk heap of a metabolism will turn into a race car. It'll kick into gear, and those tight jeans will be falling off your hips.

In other words, if you've spent the last year eating ice cream and cheeseburgers, your metabolism isn't to blame—it's the fact that you've eaten more calories than you've burned off, which has slowed down your entire system because you're carrying excess baggage.

It's time to smarten up, stop blaming, and know that anyone can lose weight regardless of their genetic programming.

SO WHY DO YOU HEAR SO MUCH ABOUT THE METABOLISM? It's true that your own unique, specific one *does* dictate how many calories your individual body will burn in one day. It's just easy science to know that you can help the situation by eating less calorie-laden foods and getting moving. Call it your own metabolism makeover.

Still confused? Let me give you more of an in-depth science lesson, but I'll be brief. Metabolism is actually the sum of all chemical processes that take place in the body as they relate to the movement of nutrients in the blood after digestion, resulting in energy, growth, release of wastes, and other bodily functions; and it takes place in two steps. The first is the constructive phase *(anabolism)*, where smaller molecules (amino acids) are converted to larger molecules (proteins). The second step is the destructive phase, *(catabolism)*—here, larger molecules (as glycogen) are converted to smaller molecules (as glucose).

Three factors determine your metabolic rate, which is the amount of calories your body uses every day: (1) the basal metabolic rate (BMR), or the rate your body uses energy for vital body processes, (2) the rate you burn energy during physical activity, and (3) the rate you use energy during digestion of food. Therefore, to improve your metabolic efficiency, *all* you need to do is change what you eat and how much you move. If you do both at the same time, I promise that you'll experience a major difference in how you look and feel.

My clients always ask me, "How can I speed up my metabolism?" It's funny, because after I give them my answer, they often have a look of disappointment on their face, but that's just the way it is. The best way to speed up your metabolism, barring any thyroid disorders, is exercise, which will help you reduce body fat and increase lean muscle mass. If you do so, your metabolism will increase and help you in the weight-loss process. Actually, a combination of both aerobic exercise and weight training is optimal for burning fat and improving your metabolism.

□——□——□

THE DOS AND DON'TS OF METABOLISM

1. *Do* weight-train. If you increase your body's lean muscle mass, it will increase your resting metabolic rate.

2. *Do* engage in aerobic activity. Get off the couch! Walk, jog, run, bike, or do any activity that gets your heart pumping. Start making aerobic exercise part of your daily routine.

3. *Do* eat more food. No, this isn't a typo. If you don't eat enough food, you'll slow your metabolism down, so be sure to eat four to six small, complete (with protein, carbohydrates, and fat), and nutritious meals throughout the day.

4. *Don't* eat junk food. Get rid of it—it's unhealthy and simply not the best choice for weight maintenance or loss. Believe me when I say with complete authority that no one ever built a six-pack of abs by making sugary or greasy foods the mainstay of their diet plan. In other words, one or two of your small meals a day can't be a cupcake or a slice of pizza, which are filled with fat, chemicals, salt, and preservatives. These are the things that mess up your system, don't allow you to digest, stop your waste processes, and end up packing on the pounds.

For the same amount of calories, you could choose a healthier snack of wheat bread, tuna, and a salad, which will burn off you quickly and actually *help* in the weight-loss process. By the way, you'll also feel much better eating healthier, and soon won't crave the junk food at all. Trust me on that one. Even my clients who were once the biggest addicts come to me and say, "Just the idea of that garbage makes me want to gag now."

5. *Do* eat frequently. Studies have shown that eating smaller, more nutritious meals every few hours aids metabolism and weight loss. And before you say anything, you *do* have the time—you're making it for your health. Later in this book, I'll even tell you about some quick and easy meals that can be prepared in no time at all, and give you recipes for handy snacks that you can take with you on the road.

6. *Don't* skip meals. Skipping meals can actually slow your metabolism down. You want to put your body on a schedule, so be sure to eat every three to four hours to keep that metabolism running high. Skipping breakfast is the worst thing you can do, because you'll mess up your metabolism for the entire day and start an onslaught of food cravings. Wake up 15 minutes earlier and eat—it's worth it.

7. *Do* keep yourself hydrated. Drinking water throughout the day is an extremely important metabolism tool: It keeps your major organs running at top speed, washes away impurities in your system, and helps flush fat. I'm sorry to say that Diet Coke doesn't have the same effect. Many people have told me that they hate water, but I promise that *you'll* love what it does for you. Just keep a chilled bottle of it on your desk and sip every now and then until it's gone. When you're thinking about how much you hate water, think about how sipping is so much easier than running another five miles.

8. *Do* get enough sleep. Lack of sleep will result in your body's inability to recover from exercise, and you won't have as much energy to perform daily activities or exercise. Your solid eight hours a night is a little "assist" to your workout. Just like your iPod, you need to recharge, or there will be no power.

9. *Do* drink tea and eat spicy foods. Studies have shown that green tea is a good metabolism stimulator, as is spicy food such as wasabi mustard. I love the taste of both and try to incorporate them into my diet whenever I can.

10. *Do* consume sports drinks. There are numerous metabolic stimulators on the market that contain ingredients (such as green tea) that will help assist in boosting your metabolism. Try your local health-food store for some of these drinks, but please check with your doctor first to see if they're a healthy alternative for you.

Now that you're more familiar with your metabolism, let's work on changing your eating habits.

CHAPTER 3

THE **TRUTH**
EATING PLAN

My diet isn't a strict one that's impossible to follow . . . cheating is even involved. I'm like everyone else in that there are days when I fall off the healthy-eating wagon, so I've found that any good plan needs a cushion to break our fall and make sure that we don't start a never-ending downward slide.

My philosophy as a trainer is that we need to build in these "cheats" so that we don't feel like failures if we eat a cookie. I don't believe in cheat *days,* but cheat *meals.* I've found that entire days mess up our metabolism to the point that it's really hard to get back on track. One cheat meal will have little to no effect on our progress, but it will work wonders for our mental status.

Oh, the other good news about my eating program is that it's an easy, not-at-all complicated plan that won't make you feel deprived.

Before we begin, I'd like to give you a quick nutrition lesson. Please don't skip this part (I know my clients!), because it's valuable information that will help you stick to your diet plan.

A QUICK NUTRITION LESSON

Protein, carbohydrates, and *fats* are the three categories of food nutrients that come into play when you start to examine what you've been eating—and why you've gained weight and how you plan to lose it. It's crucial that you understand exactly what these three components of nutrition do for your body. I know you've heard that in order to shed pounds, you need to stop eating carbohydrates. That's not entirely true, and before you drop an entire category of food, it's important to know the function of each nutrient group.

Let me go ahead and break them down for you:

1. Protein. This is the most important nutrient of all because it's the only one that actually feeds the lean muscle tissue in your body. If you don't eat enough protein, then you're going to lose lean muscle tissue. If you're trying to achieve a toned or muscular physique, it will be virtually impossible to do so without consuming protein.

Have you ever glanced at someone who's lost a lot of weight by restricting protein intake? They look like a smaller version of themselves, but with the same amount of flab. (By the way, I call that "the flubber look." We don't want flubber, do we?)

2. Carbohydrates. *Carb* has become the new four-letter word in the dieting world. Carbohydrates are supposedly the bad guys these days, with bread as public enemy number one. Yet most people have been misinformed about this nutrient group. So before you start to drastically reduce your carb intake because your friend lost five pounds on the "New York, New York Diet" (or whatever) let me remind you that carbs are necessary to the human body.

Carbohydrates provide the most easily accessible energy source for your system. Without any in your diet, your body is forced to use an alternative, less-efficient source that won't give you the same jolt of electricity. This is the reason why if you restrict carbs, you're guaranteed to feel tired and weak all the time. A young mom who came to me, for instance, explained how she actually passed out in the gym after a workout, and the treadmill wasn't entirely to blame. It turns out that she wasn't eating any carbs and was pushing herself at work, at home, and at the gym—so her body just finally waved a white flag and said, "I surrender." By the way, carbs are also important when it comes to your brain functions.

My daily eating plan includes healthy carbohydrates. I don't eat slices of white bread, but I do incorporate healthy wheats and even pasta on occasion. Why? Well, energy, breathing, and brain functions aren't areas where I want to mess around.

Let me say it one more time: *Carbohydrates are not the enemy.* Eating too many of the wrong kinds is what gets you into trouble. You see, carbs come in two forms: simple and complex. Simple carbohydrates contain table sugar *(sucrose)* or natural sugar (*fructose,* which is found in fruit, or *lactose,* which is found in milk).

When you eat too many simple sugars, including corn syrup and a variety of concentrated sweeteners, your body produces insulin to counteract the effect. This results in a fast drop in your blood-sugar level, which will leave you feeling lethargic. That simple boost from sugar is short-lived, which is why athletes chug Gatorade during a sporting event—they want the "quick hit" burst of energy.

Complex carbs, on the other hand, are released slowly in the bloodstream, thereby providing your body with a long-burning fuel supply. There's no energy rush, and your body doesn't really get cravings for these type of foods. There's a low-energy release, and your blood-sugar level remains even, thus avoiding the roller coaster of high and low blood-sugar levels brought on by simple carbs.

The TRUTH eating plan will focus on complex carbs, with the goal being to reduce your cravings for simple sugars. I promise that over a period of time, you won't even miss the simple carbs, and it might even reach the point where they gross you out a bit.

3. Fats. This nutrient group has an even worse rep than carbs . . . but what if fats could be used as an additional energy source? What if I told you that they're crucial to the maintenance and condition of your hair, skin, and nails? Well, all of the above is true. Now this doesn't mean that you should eat an entire jar of extra-chunky peanut butter, but it *does* mean that you need to incorporate fat in moderation into your diet as an essential and helpful nutrient.

One thing to note is that all fats are not created equal. The monounsaturated and omega-3 ones found in foods such as peanut butter, nuts, seeds (including flaxseed), canola and olive oil, and fish like salmon are better choices in the fight against cardiovascular disease. They also provide essential fatty acids and fat-soluble vitamins that are required for good health. However, I'm sorry to report that the fats you find in doughnuts, candy, fried foods, and those gooey cinnamon buns available at the airport are terrible for you. These include the bad fats (or the saturated, hydrogenated, and oxidized ones) including the much-publicized evil trans-fatty acids. Keep these fats to a minimum in your diet.

Okay, now that our nutrition lesson is over, let's get right to the eating plan that will help you drop that excess weight forever.

IT'S ALL ABOUT CHOICES

There's no way that I can give you a diet plan without referencing my two previous books, *The TRUTH* and *Frank Sepe's ABS-olutely Perfect Plan for a Flatter Stomach.* It's not just that I believe in what I wrote in those works, but I also follow what I wrote in them every single day of my own life. It's also heartening for me to know that there are thousands of people out there who have made these books a way of life. I have a stack of letters in my office that document these readers' successes—and now I'd like to add one more person to that list . . . you. So let's not waste another second!

Already in this chapter, you've learned the benefits of all three nutrient groups: protein, carbohydrates, and fats. Remember that knowledge is power, and now you're aware that you need all three of these nutrients in your daily menu. (I know that there are many of you out there who haven't had all three in your daily plan in years—or maybe ever. Well, there's no time like the present to get yourself on the right eating track.)

I'm not a doctor, so if you have any further questions about nutrition, I suggest that you broach them with your health-care professional before you start on this or any other plan. But I *have* made nutrition and exercise my specialty over the last 15 years—and during that time, I've heard about every single fad diet ever invented, including the insane idea that you only eat foods that are orange. (Whoever pushed that one is probably sitting on an island somewhere, laughing and eating a cheeseburger.) Since those who follow fad diets simply get fatter and fatter every year, we know that they're just a waste of time.

My plan is different because it's not a diet—it's a new way of life that pairs nutrition with exercise. The combination will lead to fat loss and better health. It's just that simple.

THE OTHER DAY I HAD A CLIENT ASK ME, "What's the difference between someone who's successful at losing weight and someone who isn't?" It was a great question, and my answer was this: "It all boils down to choices, and the ones we make dictate how we look and feel."

In other words, if you willingly make fattening foods a part of your daily ritual, then you're making the choice to eat in an unhealthy way. And one of the side effects of that choice will be the extra padding on your waist, hips, or rear end. Similarly, if you opt for sitting in front of the TV instead of working out, then you've chosen not to fit into those slimmer jeans. You made that decision, which is your own business, but it comes with consequences.

I've had many clients who want to blame someone for the fact that they're overweight and out of shape. I always tell them the same thing: "Just because they built a doughnut shop a block from your house doesn't mean that you have to stop there every day after work. Don't go there for just one day, and prove to yourself that you can stop what's ultimately destructive behavior. I promise that you'll feel empowered by just not giving in for that one day. And guess what? Knowing that you can make the choice and be in control for one day will help you find the willpower to achieve the same results the next day. After a week or so, you'll actually say to yourself, 'I can't believe I ever went in there.'"

It's all about choices, my friends, and the good ones will have a positive effect on your body. Think of yourself as a brand-new Ferrari—would you put inferior gas into something so precious? Yes, the car still might run, but you won't get optimal performance out of it. The same goes for your body.

Just reading this book means that you've made the choice to start trying to change the way you eat. Now I want you to make up your mind and firmly decide that you're going to do what it takes to reach your physical goals.

I make the right eating choices almost every day because I owe that much to myself—and so do you. The first step is for me to outline what some good choices are, and which ones will cause you to fail.

Poor Choices for Losing Weight
(in no particular order)

- Soda (thanks to the sugar and excess calories)

- Potato chips and packaged snack foods

- Deep-fried foods

- Ice cream

- Margarine and other spreads

- Processed baked goods such as cakes, cookies, candy, and doughnuts

- Alcohol (because it's calorie dense and might cause you to make other poor eating choices)

Better Choices for Losing Weight
(in no particular order)

- Protein, including turkey, chicken, egg whites, beef (flank steak), salmon, whitefish (halibut, cod, and so forth), swordfish, fat-free cottage cheese, beans, and legumes

- Protein powers—I personally like these MET-Rx products: Original Meal Replacement and RTD 51

- Carbohydrates, including leafy green vegetables, baked or boiled potatoes, sweet potatoes or yams, brown or white rice, oatmeal or oats, and whole grains including breads and pastas

- Fats, including almonds and cashews; peanut butter; olive, corn, sesame, canola, and fish oil

POOR CHOICES		GOOD CHOICES	
BREAKFAST	Calories	**BREAKFAST**	Calories
3 eggs	225	5 egg whites	85
Hash browns	320	Oatmeal	150
Buttered bagel	400	Banana	105
Coffee with cream and sugar	100	Coffee with nonfat creamer and sugar substitute	23
LUNCH			
Ham and cheese sandwich on white bread with mayo	460	**LUNCH**	
		Turkey sandwich on rye bread with nonfat mayo	328
Candy bar	250	Apple	81
Regular cola	200	Sugar-free beverage	0
DINNER			
Chicken caesar salad	630	**DINNER**	
Dinner roll	214	Grilled chicken breast	215
Chocolate-chip cookie	190	Yam	160
Regular cola	200	Large bowl of strawberries	92
		Sugar-free beverage	0
SNACK			
1 cup ice cream	500	**SNACK**	
		1 cup strawberries	46
TOTAL: 3689		**TOTAL: 1285**	

CHEAT MEALS

I'm not saying that you have to go through your entire life without eating the higher-fat, simple-carb foods that you love, but if you want to succeed at losing weight, then you might commit to refraining from them on a regular basis. If you start a diet (although I hate that word—I prefer *lifestyle change* or *eating plan*), you must change your habits. Yet, as I mentioned earlier, this doesn't mean that you're not entitled to a cheat meal.

Let's say that you've diligently stayed on your plan for at least two weeks. But when you go to sleep, you don't dream of sneaking away with Brad Pitt or Angelina Jolie—you want to snuggle with a sizzling piece of fried chicken and caress a gorgeous slice of cheese-and-pepperoni pizza. This doesn't make you strange, but simply human. I mean, can you imagine never having freshly baked chocolate-chip cookies or a glass of good wine again? Are you supposed to go through life singing "Happy Birthday" without diving a fork into some rich, delicious cake? Come on! That just doesn't seem fair . . . or possible.

Many diets make it clear to you that you can never have your favorite things. Well, I don't know about you, but I'm not going through the rest of my life without peanut M&M's. Take a minute and look at the back of this book. Yes, this body eats M&M's, *but not every day.*

You see, one of the reasons most diets fail is because they're too restrictive—they don't allow you to ever deviate from the program, so if you do stray, the feeling of failure is overwhelming. Are you a failure if you have a plate of spaghetti and meatballs? Absolutely not. That's why I believe that everyone should schedule a cheat meal into his or her weekly nutritional plan. This means that one day a week you're entitled to have one meal of anything you want. Please reread

that sentence because you're not hallucinating. I did say "anything you want." Cheeseburger and fries? No problem. Ben &
Jerry's? Sure. That big extra-cheese pizza? Go for it.

But again, don't confuse a cheat meal with a cheat day—
one meal means *one* meal.

THIS CHEAT MEAL SERVES MANY POSITIVE PURPOSES, especially metaboli-
cally. Your body is incredibly adaptive, so when you change
your eating patterns to create weight loss, it gets used to the
new program in a very short period of time. Your body will
start to accept your new way of eating as a *maintenance* program instead of a weight-reduction plan. This translates into
your getting results for a period of time, and then the weight
loss inevitably slows down as your body adapts to this new
way of life.

I know that this is terribly frustrating, but believe it or
not, your cheat meal can actually help offset this metabolic
nightmare. When you have a high-calorie meal or a few foods
that your body isn't getting on a regular basis, you shock your
metabolism back into action. Yes, your calories for that day will
be higher than normal, but that *also* shocks your metabolism.
The key is that you must return to your diet the next day, in
order to experience a caloric deficiency from the prior day's
eating. Your body (which you've now tricked) should respond
by dropping more weight.

That's great news, but I think that there's an even better
side effect from the cheat meal: It helps you keep some sort
of normalcy in your life. If you want to go on a social outing
with your friends, family, or significant other, then you can
just make it coincide with your cheat meal. Do you have a hot
date? Congratulations! Go ahead and eat whatever you want
(except for pasta, which is always too messy for a date).

The best part of the cheat meal is that it keeps you from feeling as if you failed. In fact, I prefer to call them "*sanity* meals."

GETTING STARTED FOR WEIGHT LOSS

The worst thing you can do if you want to lose weight is just jump on the dieting bandwagon. This means that one day you're eating 18,000 calories and the next you're down to 1,500. I'm exaggerating here (at least I hope), but this is how most people fail.

Your body will physically rebel against any drastic decrease in your daily food intake. In addition, you can't *mentally* handle the extreme change. That's why our first step is for you to take a week and gradually wean yourself from your poor eating habits. Eat one burger and not two, a single cookie instead of ten, and a few pieces of candy instead of the whole bag. (Perhaps you'll even get to the point that you toss the candy aside completely and reach for an apple instead.) These are small but important changes that will help you start your real plan.

I want you to gradually start eating healthier, cut out the junk food, and begin walking to get some exercise . . . and I also want you to get out a pen.

YOUR WEIGHT-LOSS JOURNAL

You need to purchase a journal or a notebook, which will be your weight-loss log. This is a crucial part of your plan, and not because you can gnaw on it when you get hungry.

I want you to write down your goals on the first page of your journal, for example: "I want to get rid of 20 pounds so that I look great at the reunion," or "I want to drop 50 pounds by next summer, so I can go to the beach and feel great." I'd love for you to write: "I want to lose 15 pounds just so I feel better and have more energy to run around with my kids," but your goal is ultimately up to you.

Writing your weight-loss goal down makes it a real commitment that's out there to be achieved, and it also makes it easier to decide on definitive nutrition and exercise plans to help you achieve that aim. In the pages of your journal, you'll be writing down everything you eat each day, along with details about what type of workout you did. Writing this information down will help you make necessary adjustments, especially if you're at a plateau or aren't getting the most out of your program. In other words, your journal will tell you where you've been and where we're going together.

I'd also like you to find some time to write down your feelings and thoughts about the day. You might discover that you eat more when you're bored, for instance, or stress makes you reach for simple carbs. Knowing this information can help you combat those issues in the future.

There are other things that you should record in your journal. These include:

1. Body-part measurements. I want you to note how many inches around your arms, chest, waist, hips, thighs, and calves are, because you want to make sure that you're losing weight in all the right places. For example, if you lose three inches off your arms and gain an inch on your waist, then something's wrong.

2. Body-fat percentage. A test using skin calipers or that dips you in water will help determine exactly how much of your body is occupied by fat. A better way of thinking about it is you're measuring your lean body mass. I know that there are some of you who don't want to know this number, but please just do it. It's only a starting point—and it's thrilling to see that number go down as we work your plan.

By the way, the scale is a good weight-loss tool, but it's not as effective as a body-fat test. There should come a time when the number on the scale remains the same, but your body-fat levels drop. This means that you've gained lean mass, and the body-fat test is the only way to determine your progress here. (By the way, my body fat is 8 percent. I thought you might want to know, but don't hate me for it—you can get there, too.)

3. The dreaded scale. It's not your enemy anymore, but rather a tool to measure how much closer you're getting to your new life. I'd like you to weigh yourself on an empty stomach first thing in the morning, and only do it once a week. Jumping on the scale every day is self-defeating because the number can jump if you've had an extra glass of water. If you stick to once a week, you'll get a more accurate measurement of your progress without torturing yourself with the daily test.

Remember that everyone is different—your progress depends on *your* willpower and *your* body. I promise that if you stick with the plan, then the end result will be amazing for you.

PUTTING TOGETHER A SOLID PLAN

Now it's time to put together an eating program that will supply you with protein, carbohydrates, and fats that will help you lose weight. You need a plan that doesn't restrict calories too much because you don't want to lose muscle as you're losing fat. It's also important to keep in mind that the exact eating plan that works for your friend might not work for you, and vice versa. It's only through trial and error that you'll find your perfect weight-loss program. My plan is not set in stone, and I encourage you to personalize it, which will guarantee success.

Now I'm going to guide you through the formula that will determine how much you eat. Please don't get scared and think that you have to be a mathematician to figure this out. It's actually a very simple formula that will serve as your starting point. By this, I mean that you'll have to make adjustments as you go along. For example, let's say that you're very active. If you find that you're losing weight too fast, you'll need to bump up the protein/carbohydrates content. But if you're sensitive to carbs, you might choose to decrease the amount you consume.

There are numerous reasons to make changes to the formula—this is why you really need to make those journal entries, so you'll have a written record of what's working and what needs to be tinkered with. It's the only way you'll be able to move in a positive direction.

THE FORMULA FOR WEIGHT LOSS

In my first book, *The TRUTH,* I recommended a lifestyle program that included a nutritional program, weight training, and cardio. In this book, I won't go as in depth on the exercise programs—I offer a beginner and intermediate workout on the enclosed DVD that will help you immensely, but for a more detailed plan, I suggest that you check out *The TRUTH.*

Anyway, when I put together my first book, I took into consideration the amount of cardio and weight training you'd be performing. Thus, I suggested a formula of:

1 gram of protein per current body weight
1 gram of carbohydrates per current body weight
.22 grams of fat x current body weight

Since *The TRUTH* calls for a specific type of training, I allowed for a higher percentage of calories. However, you might find that you need a different formula because of the specific exercise program you're following. If you're still using the plan from *The TRUTH,* then follow the formula I listed above because I know it's working. You can refine it based on information you garner on the following pages.

THE *NEW* FORMULA

The following eating program is one that I strongly believe in, and it has helped thousands of people who have used it to great success.

Basically, it's the same formula as above, except you're using your *target* body weight as a starting point. (If you have a really high metabolism and are working out as hard as you can, then you may need to increase your caloric intake.) Therefore, the new formula is:

1 gram of protein per target body weight
1 gram of carbohydrates per target body weight
.22 grams of fat x target body weight

WHAT IS TARGET BODY WEIGHT?

Your target body weight is what you're striving to achieve and then maintain for the rest of your life. I'd like you to be realistic about this number—if you're 400 pounds and want to weigh 120, for instance, your caloric intake will be too drastic of a change. Your target weight should be within reason.

If you weigh 200 pounds and your target is 175, then that's a realistic change. You should check with your doctor before starting this or any other program, especially if you need to lose more than 100 pounds. If you need to lose more than 100 pounds, then you should definitely consult with your doctor or a medical professional who specializes in safe weight loss. Once you reach your target weight, then redo your formula to strive toward your next goal.

Here are a couple of examples:

Male

>Current weight: 220 pounds
>Target weight: 200 pounds
>Daily protein intake: 200 x 1 = 200 grams
>Daily carb intake: 200 x 1 = 200 grams
>Daily fat intake: 200 x .22 = 44 grams
>**Total calories** = 1,996

(**Note:** Carbs and protein equal four calories per gram, while fat equals nine calories per gram.)

Female

>Current weight: 135 pounds
>Target weight: 125 pounds
>Daily protein intake: 125 x 1 = 125 grams
>Daily carb intake: 125 x 1 = 125 grams
>Daily fat intake: 125 x .22 = 27 (round off) grams
>**Total calories** = 1,243

THE NEXT STEP

Losing weight isn't easy because you have to really pay attention to the details. This can be inconvenient at times, but trust me when I say that the work will become a distant memory when you finally slip into those European-cut blue jeans in a size usually reserved for the woman on the cover of the current issue of *Us Weekly*.

To get to that place, you first need to find out how much you're eating. This is an easy task because of nutritional labels, which are very comprehensive these days. Here are a few tips that will help you stay on your formula:

1. Do a little research before you fill your plate. Purchase an inexpensive book that breaks down the grams of certain foods, and write down the nutrient content of the foods you eat. This type of book will make your life a whole lot easier because it will detail how many grams of protein, carbs, and fats are in a particular food.

2. It also helps to prepare each day's meals the night before. Weigh each item on a food scale so that you can be exact. As time progresses, you'll know the grams of most foods from memory—but in the beginning, the scale will help ensure that you're eating correctly.

If you're going to be eating out, you can't measure your foods, so you have to just guesstimate. If you have a plate in front of you, it should be cut into three equal parts, consisting of vegetables, a protein (such as chicken, fish, or beef), and a carb (a potato, for instance).

If you're eating out, you can also use the fist method: When you measure your food by the size of your fist, one serving of protein and carbs usually equals one fist. You can also imagine a deck of cards: One serving of carbs or protein should be no bigger than a deck of cards.

3. Sports-nutrition take-out drinks have the nutritional breakdowns on the back of their products, and are great to use, especially if you're running around and can't find anything healthy to eat that fits your requirements. I usually have one on hand so that I'm not tempted to make poor choices.

FRANKLY SPEAKING: Don't be afraid of measuring your food by grams—in a matter of a week, it will become second nature to you. I could do it in my sleep by now.

MEAL PLANNING

When you start putting your nutritional program together, it helps to mentally throw out the good old days of eating three square meals a day. Your mother might not agree, but this way of eating isn't the ideal way to lose weight or maintain a healthy body.

You need to eat a minimum of four times a day—preferably even more. That's because consuming small, frequent meals throughout the day (usually every two or three hours) will help keep your blood-sugar level more consistent, deter hunger, and stop binge eating. These consistent meals will also help convince your body that you're not starving to death—and in return, your body won't hang on to your fat, but release it . . . and you'll lose weight.

The bottom line is that you need to eat to lose weight. Isn't that the best news you've heard all week?

WHAT CONSTITUTES A MEAL?

Whenever I tell people that they need to eat four or five times a day, they usually freak out in a major way, insisting, "Frank, I can't eat that much!"

What these individuals don't realize is that although they're only having two or three meals a day, they're currently snacking all the time. I have a friend who ate three square meals a day, for instance, but she continually nibbled on nuts and licorice between her meals. And when I asked her to write down everything she ate in a day, it turned out that she was adding 800 calories from her "non-meals."

When I say to eat four or five times a day, I don't mean that you have to make yourself Thanksgiving dinner with all the trimmings each time. (In fact, please don't do that!) You can have smaller snacks and protein shakes, too. I generally drink two or three protein shakes and eat three food meals on a daily basis. The shakes are great for me because they fit right into my plan—they're high in protein while remaining low or moderate in carbs and fat. I'm sure that you'll easily find a flavor that fits into your program. Oh, and if you think that a shake will make you fat, then consider that a candy bar contains many more calories—and is much, much smaller!

Now, let's put it all together and create a couple of sample meals, based on our male and female friends from earlier in the chapter:

MEAL BREAKDOWN #1
(Male, current weight: 220 pounds
Target weight: 200 pounds)

Each Meal

Protein: 50 grams
Carbs: 50 grams
Fat: 11 grams

SAMPLE MEAL PLANS

Meal 1

Protein: 4 egg whites made into an omelette
with 4 oz. chicken breast = 44 grams

Carbs: 1 cup oatmeal with 3 tbsp. raisins = 50 grams

Fat: 1 tbsp. peanut butter = 12 grams

Meal 2

Protein: 6 oz. turkey breast = 48 grams

Carbs: 2 slices rye bread and 1 medium apple = 54 grams

Fat: 1 tbsp. almond butter = 10 grams

Meal 3

Protein: 6 oz. chicken breast = 48 grams

Carbs: 1 cup baked sweet potatoes and some green veggies = 50 grams

Fat: 1 tbsp. peanut butter = 12 grams

Meal 4

Protein: MET-Rx (my choice) or any other protein powder = 50 grams

Carbs: 8 oz pineapple juice and 2 rice cakes = 50 grams

Fat: .7 oz peanuts = 10 grams

(You can adjust meal breakdown for 5–6 additional meals.)

MEAL BREAKDOWN #2
(*Female, current weight:* 135 pounds
Target weight: 125 pounds)

Each Meal

Protein: 31 grams
Carbs: 31 grams
Fat: 7 grams

SAMPLE MEAL PLANS

Meal 1

Protein: 1 scoop protein powder = 30 grams

Carbs: 1 cup oatmeal with 1 cup strawberries = 32 grams

Fat: ½ tbsp. peanut butter = 6 grams

Meal 2

Protein: 4 oz. turkey breast = 32 grams

Carbs: 2 slices rye bread = 32 grams

Fat: .5 oz. almonds = 8 grams

Meal 3

Protein: 4 oz. chicken breast = 32 grams

Carbs: 1 cup rice = 25 grams

Fat: .5 oz. cashew butter = 7 grams

Meal 4

Protein: 4 oz. halibut = 28 grams

Carbs: 1 cup lettuce and 1 cup broccoli with 2 tbsp. fat-free dressing = 30 grams

Fat: 2 oz. olives = 8 grams

(Adjust meal breakdown for 5–6 meals.)

ADJUSTING YOUR PLAN

Remember that what I've outlined here is just your starting point, and if you have a really high metabolism and are working hard in the gym, then you need to increase your caloric intake.

You'll also be able to tweak your program as time progresses, keeping a close eye on how your body reacts to the daily food intake. Give yourself a two-week period on the original plan so that your body can adapt to the diet and then make the necessary adjustments. For example, let's say that you're following the plan and have completed six hours of cardio a week . . . and you've already lost ten pounds. This is a little too dramatic for long-term success, so I'd slow it down a tad by adding some more protein and carbs to your intake.

If you're an athlete who plays a particular sport, then perhaps you might need more carbohydrates for performance. You could also be someone who's carb sensitive, so it's possible that you'll choose to lower your intake of them and raise your protein quota. Just make the necessary adjustments until you reach a point where you're losing weight and feeling great—the combination of both of those elements will ensure your long-term success. And you'll suddenly realize that you're not on a "diet" anymore; you've simply adopted a new, healthier way of living.

TIME TO PICK YOUR MEALS

Now that you know your personal nutrient requirements for each meal, it's time to pick the foods you'll be consuming. Everyone likes variety in an eating plan, which is why I want you to choose items that are healthy, normal, and easy to find in every supermarket in the world. No wild-boar burgers on my plan, thank you very much.

Here's an example of how it works. Let's say that you're supposed to eat 50 grams of protein per meal. Simply go to the TRUTH Master Food List (see page 157) and choose the protein source that you want to eat. Chicken is always an excellent choice, since it has about eight grams per cooked ounce—if you eat six ounces, your protein requirement is complete for that meal. (Yes, I know that this is only 48 grams of protein and not 50, but you don't have to be exact. Just make sure you're within a couple of grams and you'll be fine.)

You also need to get in your 50 grams of carbs per meal. If you're in the mood for a sweet potato, I've got news for you: One cup has 48 grams, so that will certainly satisfy your carb needs for that meal. And don't forget that you absolutely need to have a little fat—about 11 grams. One tablespoon of peanut butter will give you what you need.

We've just created a meal that's not only tasty, but also complete and satisfying. Mission accomplished! But don't take this sample meal and repeat it daily or you'll get very bored. Let your fingers do the walking to the Master Food List and circle those foods that you enjoy. Play with the math a little bit and create meals that will keep you happy, healthy, and on track.

THE NEXT CHAPTER should help answer any additional questions you may have about weight loss.

CHAPTER 4

WEIGHT-LOSS Q & A

Just in case I haven't been 100 percent clear on this subject, this chapter presents some of the questions I'm most frequently asked by my clients. I hope that my responses will help you, too.

Question: "So, this sounds pretty great—I can just eat right, lose weight, and never exercise, right?"

Frank says: Ah, if only it were that simple. I hate to tell you, but the only real way to lose excess body fat is to combine your eating program with both weight training and cardiovascular exercise. These three major components work synergistically to burn fat.

You should follow a full-body routine, lifting weights that are heavy enough to stimulate new muscle growth, a minimum of three days a week (four would be ideal, but I'm trying to be realistic here). And I don't want you to just go through the motions—you need to train hard and with the gusto that I know you've been storing up inside of you for years.

As far as cardio is concerned, you absolutely can't remove this component from the mix. Again and again I hear from clients that they hate to do cardio. Now *you* don't have to love it, but you must do it. I suggest that you mix up working out indoors and outdoors—Rollerblade, jog, or use a StairMaster four days a week. I'd also like you to stay active on days when you aren't formally doing cardio. On those "off days," you can ride your bike, take a long walk with your dog, or grab your mate and go play tennis . . . just get out there and move a little bit. (Reaching for the remote control doesn't count.)

You can check out my first book, *The TRUTH,* for five levels of weight training and a number of cardiovascular workouts. I've also provided a special DVD in this book that includes a beginner weight-training program that you can do at home or at the gym three times a week for a full-body workout. (I've also included an intermediate program on the DVD that can be done at your gym.) The first week of any exercise plan is always tough, but grit your teeth and get through it. You might even find yourself looking forward to your workouts. (No, I haven't gone crazy here).

Question: "How do I lose weight quickly?"

Frank says: That's the big question, isn't it? The food and fitness industries have made billion of dollars coming up with pseudo-solutions to this one, but now it's time to talk turkey (an excellent protein, by the way). *There is no fast track to permanent weight loss.*

I'll give you a moment to digest that and realize that common sense is your first tool when it comes to working on your body. Yes, you can drop some "water weight" or even a few pounds quickly, but research shows that people who do so are more than likely to put it all back on. The truth is that anyone can lose weight fast by reducing his or her total caloric rate to virtually nothing or doing a liquid diet—but these plans are impossible to stick with for a long period of time and will actually harm your body if you try. Please don't go for the quick fix and become a yo-yo dieter (someone who gains and loses the same pounds over and over again). Research has also shown that over the long haul, such dieters end up gaining even more weight then they lose. That sounds depressing to me.

Question: "How can I be overweight if I don't overeat?"

Frank says: It's sad that most people don't realize exactly how much they do eat in the average day. I like to coach my clients to eat four to six meals in a day, as I mentioned previously, and most of them freak out at me when I first suggest it. "Frank, I can't possibly eat that much," I hear. . . . Uh-huh.

The truth is that you *do* eat that much—you just forget about the candy bars, extra-large iced mochas, or that buttered roll that you ate at the sink while reading the mail. There was also that cookie you took off the tray at work and that half sandwich that the kids didn't want. So you're probably eating much more than you think you are, and when you combine that with little to no exercise, then that's why your pants don't zip up anymore.

I've also seen overweight people who really *don't* eat that much, but they hardly ever move and live a very sedentary lifestyle. Their calories burned don't exceed what they're eating, which is your basic formula for losing weight. Here's a quick example: Let's say that a woman needs 1,500 calories a day to maintain a reasonable weight, but she ends up taking in 1,600. That extra 100 calories a day will result in close to a ten-pound gain a year if she doesn't exercise.

Question: "I have to eat out on a regular basis for my job, plus it's a social activity for my family. Does this mean that I'll never lose the weight because menus are just too tempting?"

Frank says: The good news is that I love to eat in restaurants, too, and most of them are wise to those of us who watch what we eat. Almost every eatery I know has something healthy on it—it's up to you to ignore the triple-cheese lasagna and think, *I'm going to enjoy myself just as much by having the chicken and knowing that someday I'll have the lasagna as a special treat.*

When I'm out, I like to order grilled chicken, steak, sushi, and other fish that's not fried. Be careful of designer salads, which are often loaded with fattening cheese- and mayo-based dressings. That's not a dieting choice. Here's a suggestion: If you're running around on business, you can also skip the restaurant and supplement your diet with an RTD (ready-to-drink protein shake). I often use MET-Rx RTD 51 in similar situations.

Question: "Do I really have to start a new eating program? Aren't there any tips you can give me so that I can stick to my regular food?"

Frank says: To put it simply, there are no shortcuts to losing weight without dieting—unless you like the idea of going through liposuction. (I don't know about you, but I'd rather diet than have someone suck anything out of my body with a big machine.) There are no magic pills, and no genie in a lamp is going to pop out and grant you three wishes, including that coveted size-four dress. Even prescription weight-loss drugs and gastric-bypass surgery require you to reduce your food intake. I'm sorry, but there is just no easy way out.

Question: "Come on, Frank—how can I stick to a diet and never eat my favorite foods ever again? I might have to curl up in a corner and cry."

Frank says: Please get out of the corner. I realize that you can't banish your favorites from your eating plan. Any diet that requires you to give up something forever isn't worth the paper it's printed on. Again, this is why those low-carb diets never work, because you really can't go through life never having a piece of bread again or a bite of birthday cake. I know that if someone told me I could never eat something again, it would work on my mind day and night until my lips were attached to a box that said "Hostess" on it. . . .

I suggest a cheat meal once a week, which means that you'll never feel deprived of what you're craving for more than six days. The cheat meal will satisfy your mind while tasting great and even helping to rev up your metabolism. When you have a high-calorie meal consisting of foods that your body hasn't had on a regular basis, this can have an effect of shocking your metabolism back into action. Your calories for that day will end up higher than normal, which also kicks your fat-burning motor into gear. When you return to your diet the next day, you'll experience a calorie deficiency compared with the prior day, and your body should respond by dropping some weight. Please don't forget to exercise regularly, which will mean that the excess pounds will simply melt off.

Question: "What can I do to control my cravings?"

Frank says: We've already celebrated the idea of having a cheat meal once a week so that you don't dream about your favorite comfort food. The best way to control the rest of your cravings during the week is by not skipping any meals. Don't go for long periods without eating, and don't go on severely restricted calorie diets. If you do either of these things, it can bring upon low blood sugar, which will produce cravings for high-carbohydrate or sweet foods.

The way to combat cravings is to eat regular, complete small meals—with protein, carbs, and fats. This will help keep your blood sugar level throughout the day, which, in turn, will kill the pangs.

Question: "I lost seven pounds the first week I started dieting, but only shed one pound a week afterward. Why did my progress slow down so much? I'm depressed!"

Frank says: When you start a weight-loss plan, the first couple of weeks are like a celebration—you're dropping weight at a very rapid rate, which is exciting and encouraging. Some people will lose as much as ten pounds in the first two weeks and even drop an entire size.

But then you hit the inevitable slowing down of progress. Don't despair—this isn't the time to quit or beat yourself up mentally. The reason your body has slowed down the weight loss is because you're not losing water anymore, which is what you shed at first. Now you're losing something even better: pure fat, which comes off at a much slower pace than water weight.

I always recommend a body-fat test before starting a weight-loss program, as this will give you a true indication of just how well you're really progressing. The scale doesn't tell the whole story—notice how you're fitting into your clothes better and your face is beginning to narrow. Don't get upset if the scale isn't moving as rapidly now; after all, you're in this game to lose fat and not merely water, right? Just stay the course and focus on eating right and moving, moving, moving.

PART II

THE **TRUTH** ABOUT WEIGHT GAIN

INTRODUCTION TO PART II

I know that there are many of you out there who want to shed a few pounds, which is why you've embraced Part I of this book, so I'm trying to imagine your reaction right now. You've just flipped to this chapter, read the title of Part II . . . and passed out on the rug.

Just the words *weight gain* make many run for the hills or hit the treadmill. And if I said them in Hollywood, I'd probably evacuate half of the city. But let's just calm down here. Have a glass of water, a complex carb or two, revive yourself, and know that if weight loss is your goal, then this is *not* the section for you. You need to skip it and move on to the third part of the book, which covers muscle building.

However, there are those individuals out there who will find the next few chapters to be life changing in the best possible sense. Now, while many clients tell me that those who are too thin have "no real right to complain because they've clearly got it made," that simply isn't true. These people are just as unhappy with their bodies as overweight people are, which causes them feelings of anxiety and low self-esteem. They have problems buying clothing, showcasing their bodies, going to the beach in a swimsuit that's falling off, and even letting a lover see them naked for the first time. (There are also health risks that stem from being too thin, which I'll discuss in Chapter 6.)

This next part is a very specialized part of my program for those of you who jump on the scale in the morning and hope to have gained a few pounds. You put on your Levi's and see them sagging while wishing that you had more of a body to mold.

I know that you need the same kind of assistance in your daily program that people who need to lose weight require. So I have a plan that will change your life and increase the size of your body in an attractive, healthy way.

Rest assured that my program isn't about extreme muscle building or developing a form that could get you a spot with the World Wrestling Federation. Rather, this part is for those of you who want to add some weight and do it slowly and steadily, which are always the best ways.

CHAPTER 5

WHAT IS SKINNY, ANYWAY?

It's funny that we live in a society where the mere mention of wanting to bulk up causes jaws to drop. Weight loss seems to be nirvana, as every celebrity these days seems to share his or her "current way to shed the pounds" on talk shows, in magazines, and on their Websites.

It's a lonely world for those out there whose bodies just can't seem to keep any weight on them. Their chubby friends who need to shed some pounds are constantly telling them, "Boy, I wish I had your problem." Or they've spent a lifetime hearing, "Gosh, you're so lucky—you can eat anything you want and not gain a thing."

Well, try saying that to a high school kid who can't make a team because he's thin and embarrassed that his body never "filled out" like the rest of the guys. Try relating those sentiments to a young woman like my client Jenna, whose body at age 30 resembled that very teenage boy. "Frank, I could shop in the young men's department," she told me, shaking her head. "I have no curves, no muscle definition, no stomach, no butt. Basically, I look like I'm 13, which is not so cute at this age."

Jenna had thought that she'd pack on the pounds by eating a lot of bread, butter, pasta, cookies, and ice cream . . . and her skin broke out, her hair looked dull, and she felt pretty awful. She even gained a little fat in her stomach, which is exactly what she didn't want. Who wants to look like a flat board with a pouch in front?

"My problem is just as bad as someone who needs to lose 50 pounds," Jenna told me.

I know that if Kirstie Alley were to read this, she probably couldn't understand because she's literally worked her butt off trying to slim her backside. But *I* felt Jenna's pain. You see, I was a skinny teenager with rubber-band arms and no tone before I discovered my father's basement gym, started lifting weights, and then incorporated a healthy-eating plan that developed my body in all the right—and lasting—ways.

It was a victory to shed my string-bean image. Having to work hard to develop my body was one of the first goals I met in my young life. That very personal victory was a triumph because it taught me that with a lot of hard work, anything was possible . . . including becoming a new person.

SKIN AND BONES

We've all heard someone claim that they're too thin, but how can we tell that for sure? Yes, it's easy to spot a girl who looks anorexic or lament a young man's "awkward phase," but the question remains: What is too skinny? Is it a seven-foot basketball player who weights 200 pounds? What about that size-zero woman in your Pilates class who's so thin that everyone whispers that they can see her ribs through her Lycra outfit? I know a man who actually buys children's belts because his waist is too small to shop in the "big guys'" section. (By the way, he always lies and says that he's buying the belt for his son because he's so embarrassed.) Is *he* too skinny?

The truth is that all of these people—or none of them—could have a problem with their narrow form. It's all in the way they're perceived.

Skinny has been defined as "having unattractive thinness." That makes me wonder, *Hmm. . . . If that's actually the current definition, then why are so many folks trying to become as thin as possible?* The easy answer is that people aren't actually trying to become skinny—they're trying to achieve a leaner look. You see, no one wants to have the bones in their back piercing through their shirt because their body is devoid of all fat. And very few people want to appear as if they're ill, which is what extreme thinness often conveys. (Along these same lines, someone who's trying to bulk up isn't looking to become a sumo wrestler.)

If you believe that you should gain weight, I highly doubt that you want to gain *fat.* So, in this part of the book, I'll help you increase lean muscle mass—not just some blubber for the sake of moving the scale up a few pounds. No promises. In addition, we won't put all of the new weight in one place, such as your abdomen or hips, because who wants a body that's out of balance?

Now I have to give you a quick warning: If you try to gain weight in a haphazard way, then it's very easy to pack it all on in one section, and you'll find that you have the problems of someone who needs to lose weight. So please don't get caught in this vicious cycle (and you won't if you follow my plan).

First, let me tell you why you need to get on a program in the first place . . . just turn the page.

CHAPTER 6

THE DANGERS OF BEING UNDERWEIGHT

It's not like you're actually going to fall through a bench slat or blow away in the wind. Of course seriously skinny people have heard all the jokes, including the one that "you're going to slip down your bathtub drain." Or, "You're so scrawny that you have to run around the shower in order to get wet." Or, "You're so anorexic that you make Olive Oyl look like she needs to go to Weight Watchers."

There's no sympathy for the underweight because more than half of all Americans are *over*weight. Those who need to drop a few pounds think that really thin people can simply remedy their situation by eating a couple of extra meals. If only it were that easy.

Being underweight is no laughing matter—in fact, there are real health dangers associated with it. You might be depriving your body of proper nutrition, and if so, there will be extreme consequences. Not having enough "meat on your bones" can lead to heart problems, headaches, dizziness, and even passing out. You need to speak to your doctor for a full list of all the consequences, but *I* can tell you that one of the biggest signs that you're not eating enough or aren't eating properly is weakness or fatigue.

I've had clients tell me, "Frank, my body has always been on the fragile side, and that's why I have no zip. I can barely get out of bed in the morning, and I'm too weak to do an entire workout. It's just part of my constitution."

It's dangerous to believe that this isn't a big deal—because it's actually a huge one. This type of fatigue might signify that these individuals have more serious health concerns going on within their bodies, including electrolyte imbalances, vitamin and mineral deficiencies, malnutrition, or even dehydration. Imbalances in any of these areas could lead to severe medical problems, including death, if not corrected by a physician.

HOW DO YOU KNOW IF YOU NEED TO GAIN WEIGHT IN THE FIRST PLACE?

I know that "thin is in," so why would anyone want to gain weight? Let's remember that having a great body isn't about being skinny (or fat) or having muscles on top of muscles. Each person should strive to be a *healthy* individual who follows a solid eating and exercising program that makes him or her feel good from the inside out.

One great way to know if you need to gain weight is to just ask your doctor. He or she might tell you that there are several reasons to do so:

— **For your health.** There are several medical conditions that can cause you to become underweight. If you have a problem digesting your food or suffer from persistent diarrhea, stomach pains, acid reflux, or other gastroinstestinal disorders, then seek professional help right away. Your doctor or health-care professional will be able to quickly tell you if you'd be healthier with a few more pounds on your frame.

— **To enhance your self-esteem.** Just as an overweight person might not like the way his or her body looks in the mirror, the underweight man or woman can experience the same kind of feeling each day. You may hate the way you look in jeans or in a bathing suit, and perhaps you avoid health-club locker rooms. Nor do you care for the worried looks from friends who tell you, "Why, you're just skin and bones!"

— **For self-defense purposes.** People who are very skinny have historically been considered easy marks for those who are bigger. Maybe you were pushed around in the school yard, and now you're knocked aside in the rush for people to get on the subway. In our culture, *underweight* can be synonymous with *wimpy*. This usually isn't a big problem if you're a thin woman, but if you're a skinny man, you may feel the need to try to build up your body so that you can establish more of a strong presence in this world.

— **To attract the opposite sex.** Let's say that you're single and are trying to attract a date. There's a lot of competition out there, so you want to put your best body forward. Many women want to meet a guy who has a more developed body; maybe it's that Hollywood image of a damsel feeling safe in a bigger man's embrace. If the guy has arms that are smaller than the gal's, well, it might not be her idea of a dream date. Of course, you can't measure a relationship by body types—after all, actor Adrien Brody, the superthin star of *The Pianist,* doesn't lack for dates. (Then again, he's a movie star, and there are many women who might not give his skinny self a second glance if he were just an average guy walking down the street.)

— **To participate in sports.** It's only normal to want to become bigger and stronger if you participate in sports that require more brawn. (As early as junior high school, kids have been known to try to gain weight in order to enhance their athletic performances on the field.) Certain sports even call for a certain weight. For example, if you play football and are a lineman, then you need to weigh more than the other guy who's trying to steamroll into you, and most wrestlers fight to get to a certain weight class in order to compete. If you haven't been able to make a team, then gaining some size might just get you that spot.

THE LOLLIPOP PEOPLE

There are people who are born with genes that simply burn fat like a souped-up furnace—they're on the lean side because their inner machine seems to work at a different pace. But there's a new phenomenon we're seeing these days, born of a generation that's been dieting for a lifetime, where people have *made themselves* into dangerously thin beings.

These types, which have been dubbed "lollipop people," seem to have big heads on teeny, tiny bodies that are practically skeletal—you can even see their veins sticking out. It's sad, because many of these individuals took dieting and exercising to a terrible extreme, and the result is that they've made themselves both unhealthy and unattractive. But they can't seem to stop because they live in fear of gaining an extra ounce.

The good news is that America is becoming aware of the idea that we can actually make ourselves unhealthy by over-exercising and taking dieting to an extreme. (There are even people out there who are "addicted to exercise.") If you find yourself in this category, it's time to stop, get on a solid plan, gain back a few pounds, and then develop your body in other ways that are healthy and attractive. I also recommend professional help in the form of a therapist or counselor.

Even starlets such as Paris Hilton, Mary-Kate Olsen, Kelly Ripa, Lara Flynn Boyle, and Nicole Richie have been on the receiving end of articles questioning if they need to eat a good meal. (They are beautiful women; however, I suggest that they take me up on my idea of a cheat meal every now and then!) However, let's say that the situation isn't that dire for you, but you simply need to bulk up. I know that you're out there, because when I came out with my first book, *The TRUTH*, I received many e-mails asking me why I didn't include any weight-gain plans. So that's why I added this part to the current book—I want to give you weight-gain aficionados a simple, not-at-all confusing plan that you can make a part of your daily lifestyle.

Our goals are twofold: I'll help you gain weight for health first, and to feel good about yourself second. Let's get started.

CHAPTER 7

NO LOSS—ALL GAIN

Okay, so how do you begin to gain a few pounds? The truth is that gaining the "right kind" of weight isn't necessarily an easy thing to do. It's only natural to look at tubby, greasy-burger-scarfing, carb-overloading friends and think, *Well, I'll just stuff my face and gain some pounds like they did.*

That's a very bad idea.

The same rules apply if you're overweight or underweight: Your first priority should be your health, and feeling good about how you look comes second. You're not going to achieve either of those goals by eating foods that make your system sluggish and just pack on the fat.

The last thing you want to do if you're underweight is to start eating everything in sight. I like to call this the "See-Food Diet"—basically, you eat everything you see, including fried, sugary food. The end result is that you'll likely become a rounder version of your present self . . . while also clogging your arteries, elevating your blood pressure (from all the salt), and diminishing your zest for simple things such as walking from your house to your car. You know that horrible feeling you get after a road trip where you've focused on the "four food groups": McDonald's, Burger King, Wendy's, and Kentucky Fried Chicken? Well, who wants to walk around feeling that way all the time?

If you eat everything within your grasp, you'll feel about a decade older in record time. And picture your body with 20 pounds of fat attached to it—yes, you'll look like you swallowed a basketball, which is not a trendy look (at least not the last time I checked).

THE TRUTH ABOUT THOSE WEIGHT-GAIN POWDERS

Let me tell you a quick story about a childhood friend of mine named Patrick. People in the neighborhood used to call him "The Flamingo" because he had legs that were like toothpicks.

Patrick was sick and tired of being picked on, so he bought a super-weight-gain powder that promised a whopping 1,000 calories per drink. My buddy wanted to gain some pounds quickly, so he'd dump the powder in his blender, add two huge scoops of ice cream followed by bananas, chocolate syrup, and anything else that he could find to add even more calories to the drink. (One time he threw in a jumbo-sized bag of M&M's, which was hard on his body, but even tougher on his poor blender!)

For an entire summer, Patrick drank four of these shakes every single day, which he followed with three meals of pasta drowning in gooey, melted American cheese. And even though he gained about 35 pounds in three months, he wasn't happy. All of the weight had gone directly to his gut, and he appeared to be ready to give birth to a giant beach ball. Of course, Patrick never exercised during this all-you-can-eat free-for-all . . . and on his genius plan, he ate so much fat that he probably couldn't have gained any muscle even if he had worked out.

"What should I do?" Patrick wailed to me one day. "I finally gained some weight, but I've never felt so awful in my life. It's like I can't even get through the day—I just want to nap all the time."

The moral of the story is simple: You need to be *smart* about what kinds of food you put in your body, no matter what your goal is when it comes to your shape. And don't think for one second that just because you need to gain weight I'm going to skip telling you that exercise is a must. Taking in extra calories while living a sedentary life is never the best way to achieve your health goal.

In the next chapter, I'll show you how you can incorporate exercise into the program and achieve amazing body-sculpting results. One word of caution: Please don't confuse upping your food intake and exercise with bodybuilding. If you want to get to that level, then by all means check out Part III, which deals with smart ways to build muscle. But let's not get too far ahead of ourselves. Right now, the mission is to help you gain weight in the form of lean muscle, which, when done in a slow way, is the most effective weight-gain program on the planet.

CHAPTER 8

THE **TRUTH**
WEIGHT-GAIN PLAN

There are medical reasons to gain weight that, combined with self-esteem issues, make it a smart choice (or even a necessity) for many people. However, it's not always an easy process, and you might get discouraged when the scale doesn't seem to be moving in the right direction. You may even go down a few pounds and want to throw in the proverbial gym towel. Yet just like a weight-loss program, the key is *consistency*—stick with it, and you'll see amazing results. What you want probably won't happen overnight, but think of building up your body as constructing a brand-new house: one piece at a time. In this case, it's one bite and one workout at a time.

There will be certain obstacles on your road to success that I want you to keep an eye out for while you follow the plan that I'm about to give you. For example, watch out for excessive exercise, stress, depression, skipping meals, and other poor eating habits and food choices. If you find yourself falling into any of those traps, stop, take a deep breath, and reevaluate your daily program.

Finally, remember that you can do it. Just follow the plan in this chapter, and before you know it, the body you've always imagined will be gaining on you.

IS ALL WEIGHT GAIN EQUAL?

My plan is a simple way to add lean weight to your body, not just fat. I do realize that most people don't want to be overly muscular to the point of looking freakish, but I don't plan on turning you into a bodybuilder. We're simply going to leave the land of the underweight and attain a normal and healthy frame . . . and the only way to do so is to add lean body mass instead of fat. Now, please don't freak out when you hear the word *muscle,* since gaining a little brawn will actually help shape the body that you've always wanted to call your own.

I remember going to a Yankees game last summer and seeing a guy who weighed about 225 pounds of rock-hard muscle, with veins on top of veins. He walked by a group of people who looked as if they'd just spent the last 24 hours in a doughnut shop, and they proceeded to order a bunch of beers and yak about how gross the guy looked. They spent ten solid minutes ripping the guy's body, and most of the insults were hurled by a woman who admitted that she hadn't seen her original chin since high school. The man sitting next to her—who had more rolls than an Italian bakery—piped in that the guy looked like a goon.

When did having muscles become socially unacceptable, and even worse than being obese? My point of view is "to each his own." The brawny guy in question wanted to bulk up, and he worked hard toward that goal. That isn't what I'm going to be teaching *you,* though—instead, I'm going to help you sculpt your already-slim frame into something spectacular.

If you're still worried about getting too pumped, let me give you a few more specifics. Someone who's strikingly muscular, like the man I saw at the baseball game, got that way because he was eating a special kind of diet. He was also following a very specific weight-training program that probably focused on low reps of heavy weights—which is exactly what we *won't* be doing in this chapter. I just want to get you, my thin friends, to a healthier weight.

KEEP IN MIND THAT IF YOU ONLY WEIGH 100 POUNDS and exist on junk food, then you'll have the same health problems as a heavier person. And even though you're thin, you could still have a high body fat percentage (BFP).

Bad fats will lead you to an early grave, which is why all of us need to put down the pizza and pick up a turkey wrap. The best way to gain lean body mass is to follow a nutritional plan that has a high enough caloric count so that it will feed your muscles. You want to eat complete meals that contain all three food nutrient groups: protein, carbohydrates, and fat. You'll also need to follow a weight-resistance program, because nothing will help you build muscles faster.

Now you might be thinking, *Hey, Frank, if my goal is to gain lean body mass by working out, then isn't this considered muscle building—and shouldn't I just turn to Part III?* My answer is that you're partially correct: Your muscle building will first help you return to a normal weight and then develop a strong, muscular body. If you want to take it further, then by all means, keep going to Part III. But remember that you have to crawl before you can walk!

The most important aspect of starting a weight-gaining plan is to take it step-by-step. In this chapter, I'm going to give you a starting point, and then, through trial and error, you'll personalize the nutritional plan as you get to know your body better through how you feel and your journal entries.

THE SMART PLAN FOR HEALTHY WEIGHT GAIN

The formula I'm about to outline has worked for numerous underweight clients of mine—but first, I want to go back and detail the three vital building blocks of nutrition.

1. Protein. You'll need to have an ample supply of protein in your plan if you intend on building muscle, since it's the only nutrient that actually feeds the lean muscle tissue in your body. So if you don't make protein part of your daily eating program, you're never going to gain lean muscle mass—and your body will just become a fatter version of itself. (We even have a category for these types of people in the fitness world and call them the "skinny fat people.") Let me say it one more time: *Protein builds muscle.*

2. Carbohydrates. If you're trying to obtain lean mass and create a healthier body, then you absolutely need to consume carbohydrates. The worst thing that someone who's trying to gain weight can do is not consume this nutrient, since it provides the most easily accessible energy source for your body. Without enough carbs in your diet, your body will use an alternate, less efficient path that won't give you the same energy and will leave you tired and weak.

3. Fat. You can't shun fat in your diet, but remember that not all of it was created equal. The bad kind is lurking in ice cream or doughnuts, and you need to eat the good kind. Remember to stick with monounsaturated and omega-3 fats found in foods such as peanut butter, nuts, seed, flaxseeds, and canola and olive oils.

STARTING-POINT FORMULA FOR WEIGHT GAIN

1 gram of protein per current body weight
2 grams of carbohydrates per current body weight
.20 grams of fat x current body weight

Here are a couple of examples:

<u>Male</u>

> *Current weight:* 200 pounds
> *Daily protein intake:* 200 x 1 = 200 grams
> *Daily carb intake:* 200 x 2 = 400 grams
> *Daily fat intake:* 200 x .20 = 40 grams
> **Total calories** = 2,760

<u>Female</u>

> *Current weight:* 125 pounds
> *Daily protein intake:* 125 x 1 = 125 grams
> *Daily carb intake:* 125 x 2 = 250 grams
> *Daily fat intake:* 125 x .20 = 25 grams
> **Total calories** = 1,725

(**Important notes:** Please check with your doctor before using this or any other program. If you suffer from an eating disorder, then please seek medical help from a licensed medical practitioner. Carbs and protein equal four calories per gram, while fat equals nine calories per gram. Also, you can adjust your protein up or down a notch based on the formula that I detailed above for you—pay attention to how your body reacts with 1 gram x your current body weight.)

WEIGHT GAIN FOR ATHLETES

There are very few 200-pound people out there who are considered underweight. However, there are probably some guys who are trying to bulk up in order to make the football or wrestling team. For example, I remember an athlete named Shawn Bradley who was more than seven feet tall and needed to gain weight in order to play pro basketball. This isn't a typical situation, but if it's the case for you, then you need to design a specific nutritional plan that takes into consideration a few important elements.

If you're trying to gain weight for a sport, then you're most likely practicing every single day, including weight training, cardio, and performing a whole host of other activities. All of these burn calories and must be taken into consideration when you're designing your program.

I've given you a starting point with the meal breakdowns, but this is a unique situation where every element must be factored in. So if you practice in the morning, then you need to take in more carbohydrates before you train; or if you have classes during the day or live in a dorm room, then you'll have to rely more heavily on sports nutrition for convenience. Take a look at the sample plans for the 125-pound person, and then read Part III on muscle building—this should help you put together a personalized program that fits your unique, individual needs.

MEAL PLANNING

When you start putting your nutritional program together, just throw out the notion of eating three square meals a day. Rather, you need to eat a minimum of *four* times a day—preferably even more. That's because consuming small, frequent meals throughout the day (usually every two or three hours) will help keep your blood-sugar level more consistent, deter hunger, and stop binge eating.

Now, when I say to eat four or five times a day, I don't mean that you have to make yourself a seven-course meal. You can have smaller snacks and protein shakes (in fact, I usually drink two or three protein shakes and eat three food meals on a daily basis).

Now, let's put it all together and create a couple of sample meals:

MEAL BREAKDOWN
(Current weight: 125 pounds)

Each Meal

Protein: 25 grams
Carbs: 50 grams
Fat: 5 grams

(**Note:** Estimations don't have to be exact—get as close as you can.)

SAMPLE MEAL PLANS

Meal 1

Protein: 6-egg-white omelette with 1 oz. turkey = 27 grams

Carbs: 1 cup Cream of Wheat; 1½ cup cantaloupe = 51 grams

Fat: 1 oz. avocado (trimmed) = 5 grams

Meal 2

Protein: MET-Rx Whey Powder (or any other whey protein powder), mixed with skim milk = 25 grams

Carbs: 2 slices rye bread; ½ cup grapes = 39 grams (plus 11 grams from the milk = 50 grams)

Fat: ½ tbsp. peanut butter = 4 grams

Meal 3

Protein: 3 oz. turkey breast = 24 grams

Carbs: 1 cup baked sweet potato; green salad of lettuce and cucumber = 50 grams

Fat: 1 tsp. olive oil = 5 grams

Meal 4

Protein: MET-Rx Whey Powder (or any other whey protein powder), mixed with skim milk = 25 grams

Carbs: 1 small banana; 1 tbsp. raisins = 36 grams (plus 11 grams from the milk = 50 total)

Fat: 1/3 oz. cashew butter = 4 grams

(You can mix all ingredients in a blender for a shake.)

Meal 5

Protein: 3 oz. tuna steak = 24 grams

Carbs: 2 oz. (measure uncooked) pasta; 1 cup broccoli = 52 grams

Fat: 1 oz. green-pitted olives = 4 grams

How to Make Adjustments

Please understand that this plan is not set in stone—the formula is to be used as your starting point and as a way to develop a personalized eating plan that's exactly right for your body. I'd never recommend the same plan for everyone. Yes, it's possible for people to see results on the starting-point formula, but individual systems vary. Your body might require more carbohydrates, protein, or fat, and it's up to you to figure out what makes you feel good while gaining lean muscle weight.

Now I'd like you to refer to the weight-loss portion of this book and read the passage about the importance of keeping a food journal on page 30. In case you don't want to flip pages or are in an extra lazy mood, here are the Cliffs Notes. In your journal, you'll record everything you eat and all of your workouts. You'll also note your current body fat, weight, and body measurements. All of these things combined will help you determine what changes should be made to your diet. You should retake these measurements after 30 days on the plan and compare your new numbers to those when you started. It's also a good idea to get a second physical after those 30 days. I hope that you'll be inspired by the results if you're following the plan.

Your journal will help you know if you've gained too much weight in the first week. Let's say that you packed on ten pounds, which is way too much for a week—you'll know that certain adjustments will need to be made to both your nutritional plan and your workouts to slow down your speed. Perhaps you can cut back your protein or cut back the protein *and* the carbs. Perhaps you're not working out intensely enough or doing enough cardio to burn some of the additional food you're eating, and that's why the weight gain was so rapid. It's up to you to zero in on what's right for your body.

FRANKLY SPEAKING: No one knows your body better than you do.

How Much Weight Should You Gain?

If you're severely underweight, then you should be under a doctor's care because this will affect your health. *Please do not hesitate to make that appointment today.* For the rest of you out there who just want to put on a few pounds, the answer as to how much is up to you, but the last thing you want to do is start gaining five to ten pounds a week. It's impossible to put on that much muscle in one week, so the bulk of your new form will consist of fat and water. If you want to gain weight like that, all you need to do is drink soy sauce and pickle juice—the sodium content will blow you up like a fish. (Please do not try this at home.)

I'd advise shooting for one two-pound gain each week. But be careful of how your measure your progress—realize that the scale changes every single time you step on it. If you drink water or have a big meal, the scale will move upward, whereas when you get on it with an empty stomach or after doing cardio, it will register less weight. The bottom line is that the scale will drive you crazy, especially if you're one of those people who constantly weighs him- or herself. (I see you out there!)

You do need to keep a close eye on any significant changes through your total body evaluation that we discussed in this section. That's the only true way to measure your progress.

The Importance of Working Out

I believe that everyone should do weight-resistance exercises, including people who need to gain weight. The benefits are universal, including creating lean muscle mass and increasing your strength and flexibility—I love that my gym is even flooded with senior citizens and teenagers who are doing just that.

One warning is that if you're not eating correctly, then you're not going to get any results out of the weight-training program. Your body needs extra nutrients when you're training to help it recuperate and grow. Eating correctly will work synergistically with weight-resistance exercise to assist you in developing a healthier and fit body. It's a one-two punch. (You can get more information and sample workouts on the DVD that's included with this book.)

WHAT ARE THE BENEFITS OF WEIGHT-RESISTANCE EXERCISE?

1. Builds muscle mass and strength
2. Helps regulate metabolism
3. Increases stamina and energy
4. Strengthens tendons and ligaments
5. Aids with bone density
6. Personal appearance goes "from zero to hero"

I know that many of you may resist any form of cardiovascular exercise because it burns calories. This is true, but the catch is that I'm giving you a program where your caloric intake is enough that you don't have to shun cardio. You can also adjust your nutritional program to support a heart-healthy and mentally stimulating cardio plan.

Cardiovascular exercise isn't just about fat burning—the other benefits include lowering your blood pressure, increasing your HDLs (good cholesterol), decreasing your LDLs (bad cholesterol), and improving heart and lung functions. Cardio can also help decrease anxiety, depression, and tension.

My suggestion is that *everyone* does cardio, even you underweight folks. I don't want you to overdo it, but simply get your heart pumping by incorporating it into your routine.

MY TOP-10 WEIGHT-GAIN TIPS

1. Make your meals complete (that is, include protein, carbs, and fat).

2. Eat small, frequent meals.

3. Have a big breakfast.

4. Don't shy away from red meat.

5. Get enough complex carbohydrates.

6. Supplement with protein, meal replacement powders (MRPs), and ready-to-drink shakes (RTDs).

7. Rest.

8. Weight-train, which helps build mass and strength.

9. Cycle your calorie content.

10. Drink plenty of liquids.

INCORPORATING SPORTS-NUTRITION PRODUCTS

One of the reasons why some people are underweight is because they don't have time to eat. Many folks live very hectic lives, and they end up making food a last priority: Some of them grab high-calorie fast food when they're hungry, while others just don't eat at all.

There's no reason to skip a meal when you can easily drink an MRP, RTD, or protein drink. If you have an insane schedule, I sympathize, but there's no reason why you should miss a meal when you can have a drink that's full of vitamins and minerals . . . and all you have to do is throw one in your bag. You can just shake it up and not even have to worry about mixing ingredients or having fresh milk on you.

You can also mix a drink with your own ingredients before you leave the house and carry it in a shaker bottle. It's also easy to add additional calories to a MRP or protein shake. If you're one of those people who need more carbs, for instance, then you could combine an MRP with some yogurt and a banana. Or you could blend it with skim or whole milk instead of water for a calorie boost. Just make sure that the mix fits into the formula for your nutritional plan. There are also other kinds of shakes into which you can blend milk, fruit, and protein powder.

Don't make yourself a 2,000-calorie shake and then have just one other meal during the day—it doesn't work that way. The goal is not to miss *any* of the meals on your plan. The shakes are there to help you get in the ones that are easy to miss when you're living a hectic lifestyle. Experiment with incorporating the shakes into your diet. I promise that you'll learn to love the convenience of them.

THE NEXT CHAPTER should help lay to rest any additional concerns you have regarding weight gain.

CHAPTER 9

WEIGHT-GAIN Q & A

If you have any remaining confusion on this subject, this chapter presents some of the questions I'm most frequently asked by my underweight clients. I hope that my answers will help you as well.

Question: "My doctor is always on my case because I'm very thin. A few days ago, he told me that I needed to gain ten pounds immediately. The problem is that I detest all of the high-calorie foods he put on my weight-gain list. I just don't understand why I can't eat whatever I want, like ice cream or cake. Isn't a calorie a calorie? I'm so thin that I figure I'll never get fat. Right?"

Frank says: First of all, you need to listen to your doc. If he put you on a specific diet, then you shouldn't deviate from it. I'm sure that there are specific medical reasons why you're on this particular plan, so please don't begin to make unwise choices that could hurt your health. By the way, I've never known a doctor who advised his underweight patients to use Ben & Jerry's as a medicinal tool (although wouldn't it be a great world if this were possible?).

You need to know that not all calories are created equal. Just because you're ten pounds underweight doesn't mean that you can eat junk food until you pack on those ten. A diet high in fat and sugar will add pounds of pure flab to your frame. If you really want to discourage yourself, just imagine ten pounds of chicken fat attached to your body. It's a horrible image for anyone to mull over!

Your goal is to put ten *healthy* pounds on your body in the form of lean mass, which is the only way to create a healthy and more pleasing body. Again, if you load up on junk food, then your body will never look very appealing, and you'll feel sluggish. You might even develop the first multiple chin of your life or a stomach pouch.

I'd also advise you to get a body-fat test before you start on your doctor's program, as this is a great way to determine if you're adding lean mass or pure fat. Adding weight in the form of fat can lead to an array of health risks, including heart disease, which is why your doc probably recommended the foods on your list instead of the ones you would have *liked* him to.

Question: "My entire life, people have been harping on me to gain a few pounds. The problem is that I love eating meat and am just not into carbohydrates. In a way, I've been on low-carb plan—by choice—since I was a teenager. My question is simple: Can I gain some weight by just eating meat?"

Frank says: Too much of anything is not a good idea. One of the problems with just eating meat is that this high-protein choice converts poorly into energy when you don't eat it with enough carbohydrates. If a human being eats nothing but meat and shuns carbs, then most of the meat will be converted to energy, with a tiny amount of this digested food left for storage. You won't ever gain weight on this eating plan. Again, it's all about moderation.

Back to your question, which is simple to answer: You need to start eating a more balanced diet *including* carbohydrates, which will help you pack on some weight and provide you with more energy. I'd add some potatoes, vegetables, rice, and cereals to your daily plan.

Question: "I only eat one meal a day, and then I have a couple of snacks when I feel a little bit hungry. With my busy schedule, I just don't have time to sit down and eat three squares a day. What do you suggest I do to get more calories into my plan?"

Frank says: One of the most frequent excuses I hear from my clients, whether they want to gain or lose weight, is that they don't have time to eat. This is a tough one for me to understand. The reality is that you're not *making* the time to nourish your body, and apparently you don't plan on changing what's actually harmful behavior. *You need to give yourself a break and make the time to eat properly.* What could be more important? If you don't do so, then you won't have the energy for all those other things that are consuming your time, such as work, children, and relationships. It's all about choices in life.

My advice is to preplan three solid food meals each day. Try waking up 30 minutes early to eat breakfast and also pack a healthy lunch. This might take a little dedication and will-power, but if you make eating a priority, then you'll fit it into your daily schedule. I have a client who needed to gain weight, but he worked ten hours a day and was always moving at a frantic pace. We worked together to actually schedule his three meals a day. In between those meals, I had him drink a MET-Rx RTD (ready-to-drink) shake. Since these are prepackaged, he didn't even have to mix them—all he had to do is pull a tab and take a sip. The drinks gave my client much-needed vitamins, minerals, and nutritious calories as opposed to eating a candy bar or a muffin.

Question: "My entire body has been described as 'skin and bones.' I'm just sick of how I look and want to gain weight fast. What can I do?"

Frank says: You can easily gain weight, but we need to take the word *fast* out of your vocabulary. You want to gain the weight safely and slowly, and you need to put on *quality,* not *quantity.* If you want to achieve a body that's stronger and more desirable, then you need to make a complete lifestyle change. Before you flip the switch, it's helpful to go in with the right attitude. Know in your heart that you're not going to change overnight, so any plan that promises fast results is doomed for failure. Wrap your brain around the idea that you're changing your life *forever,* and something of that magnitude might take some time. It will also take determination, consistency, and a lot of mental strength.

The first thing you need to do is start eating more of a balanced diet, consisting of three complete meals that each include protein, carbs, and fat. You can also add MRPs (meal replacement powders) and protein shakes in between your meals. And you'll need to incorporate weight training into your program in order to increase your lean muscle mass. This resistance program will include basic compound exercises to create a basic foundation for your body. Train in a pyramid fashion by starting with light weights and high repetitions, and then increase the weight and decrease your reps on every set that follows. (*Example:* 100 pounds x 12 reps, 120 x 10, 140 x 8, 160 x 6, and so forth.) Keep your workouts brief and intense—you shouldn't lift weights more than four times a week because you need to allow your body plenty of time to recuperate, rest, and grow.

A balanced diet, plus weight training, will absolutely produce amazing results that you can sustain over your entire lifetime. That's much better than some fleeting, fast fix.

Question: "Do you have any tips on how I can add even more calories to my weight-gain program?"

Frank says: I'm not sure exactly what you're eating, but I can make some simple suggestions. Eat consistently throughout the day—that is, don't go for long periods of time between meals without food. Specific recommendations to gain weight should be based on your individual needs or what's been suggested by your doctor. However, I can offer a few broad suggestions:

1. Start by adding healthy oils (including olive) to your cooked foods, since this is a quick way to pour on some extra calories. You can also marinate your meats in olive oil or add it to your salad.

2. Nuts are a great way to increase your overall calorie content. You can easily take them wherever you go and snack on them between meals, and adding peanut butter to your oatmeal or making peanut-butter sandwiches on whole-wheat bread is a nice, healthy snack.

3. Snack on fruit such as oranges, grapes, figs, dates, raisins, bananas, or pears.

4. Avocados are a good snack because they're high in healthier fats.

5. A very easy way to increase caloric intake is to add a protein shake between meals.

6. And finally, don't forget to exercise while adding calories so that the extra food doesn't convert into fat!

Question: "I'm desperately trying to gain weight, and I started using some weight-gain powder that a friend of mine recommended. Unfortunately, I just couldn't stand the taste, and my body had a hard time digesting it. Is there any other kind of shake that I can use instead of those popular sports drinks to gain weight?"

Frank says: Not everyone is a big fan of drinking sports-nutrition drinks. I've been using them for 15 years, so I know that some are better than others. I also have clients who just can't get into the whole drink thing—they have a hard time dealing with the taste or have digestion issues.

I suggest that you haul out your blender and make your own shakes. One of my favorites for weight gain consists of skim milk, a banana, and a cup of blueberries. (You can add yogurt to it as well.) There are hundreds of different combos you can try with fruit, yogurt, and skim milk . . . just don't mix up a gallon of chocolate ice cream with caramel into the shake, because then you're only going to gain blubber and not lean muscle tissue.

Question: "How does a vegetarian gain weight?"

Frank says: This sounds like a riddle to me, but the punch line is simple: If a vegetarian wants to gain lean body mass, then he or she needs to make sure that there's enough protein on the plate.

If you're not going to eat red meat, chicken, or turkey, then you need to get your protein from eggs, lentils, beans, low-fat milk, and protein drinks. It's crucial that enough protein is incorporated throughout the day if you expect to see any lean-mass gain. You'll also need to eat an ample amount of carbohydrates, just like everyone else who wants to gain weight, and begin an exercise program.

Question: "How do I know if I'm gaining weight too fast?"

Frank says: Before you start a new eating plan, you should always do the following things:

1. Pay your doctor a visit and get a full physical. Show him or her a written copy of the diet you're going to follow (whether it's mine or someone else's), for he or she should know exactly what you're eating.

2. Take measurements of your body parts. Measure your legs, chest, arms, waist, hips, and neck, and jot those numbers down in a journal.

3. Weigh yourself and get a body-fat test at your local gym or through your doctor. Also write those numbers down in your journal.

4. The last thing you need to do is set goals, such as: "In 30 days, I hope to gain eight pounds. I'll know because I'll retake my body measurements and body-fat test, and I'll weigh myself." These numbers will tell you if you're moving in the right direction. If you've gained ten pounds and 3 percent body fat in a month, for instance, then you're eating too much fat. However, if you're up five pounds and your body fat is the same or even less than when you started, then you're moving in the right direction.

   Remember that the goal is to gain *good* weight, not fat. If you're eating doughnuts and cookies every day, then you'll gain 20 pounds of fat in a month, and that's not the way to go for long-term success.

PART III

THE **TRUTH** ABOUT MUSCLE BUILDING

INTRODUCTION TO PART III

You've been working hard on your new eating plan, and that's no easy deal. You should be extremely proud of your efforts to either lose or gain weight. But now it's time to really kick your program—and your body—into higher gear.

In this section, we all reunite with the common purpose of putting together the last piece of the puzzle: muscle building. The weight-loss part of this book is for people who want to shed some pounds, and the weight-gain portion is for individuals who want to add some healthy mass. The muscle-building chapters are for *all* those who want to perfect the body they've started to develop through their various nutritional programs to fit specific needs.

What follows isn't just for bodybuilders—it's for any of you who want to take your own physique a step above the norm or build a substantial amount of lean muscle. Keep in mind that it takes years of proper diet and exercise to look like a bodybuilder, so I promise that you won't wake up one morning and be covered in bulges and veins. But you *will* be stronger and more muscular than the average person, and you'll feel empowered. Our goal is to create sinewy, fit bodies that are strong and healthy. The size of your muscles is up to you.

I know that many of you consider cardio to be a chore, but that's not the case with muscle building, which is actually a very fulfilling, relaxing, and enjoyable way to work on your body. We'll take it slowly, and soon you'll actually look forward to these workouts. One of the great benefits is on a psychological level because there's nothing like feeling strong. It's the ultimate confidence booster.

We'll take it slowly and build you up to a program that fits your individual needs, and I promise that you'll see results that will astound you.

CHAPTER 10

MUSCLE-BUILDING 101

Too many people are under the impression that you just need to eat large amounts of food, lift a few heavy weights, and—presto change-o!—you'll instantly have a physique that even Vin Diesel would envy.

If this were true, then why aren't power lifters, football players, and wrestlers Mr. Olympia winners? Even more important, why isn't everyone walking around out there with these championship figures? I can't help but look around the streets of New York City and see people who look tired and out of shape. Why aren't they simply lifting a dumbbell to feel better?

If it were only that easy! No, you must change your *entire lifestyle* in order to create the sculpted, muscular type of body found in magazines or on ESPN. A combination of eating correctly and muscle building will get you from today's shape to one that blows your mind.

I like to equate creating a muscular body with playing baseball. To play America's favorite pastime, you need a bat, ball, and a glove. To create a muscularly toned body, you also need three components: (1) an eating plan as outlined in this book (programs that are designed to build muscle), (2) weight training to build and sculpt muscle, and (3) cardio to burn the fat off so that you can get to the muscle.

Do all three and it's a home run.

REASONS WHY MEN AND WOMEN SHOULD WANT TO BUILD A MUSCULAR BODY

1. Increase everyday, functional strength
2. Improve self-esteem
3. Jump-start natural energy
4. Lose fat (muscle efficiently burns fat)

LIFTING AWAY THE MISCONCEPTIONS

Sadly, many people are misinformed when it comes to building muscle. In fact, I've heard some pretty crazy ideas on the subject over the years. One of my favorites came from a 150-pound man named Tom who was so dedicated that he'd come to the gym seven days a week and load up the bench press with 400 pounds. He didn't see the need to warm up his muscles, but he did always ask someone to spot him so that he wouldn't get hurt (his one good idea).

Next, Tom would pump his 400 pounds . . . or at least try to. The result was usually a resounding boom because the weight would come crashing down on his chest (I can only imagine how much this hurt), and then the poor spotter would have to pull this enormous poundage off of him. Tom went through this lift-and-crash routine until no one in the gym would spot him anymore. One day I approached him and asked, "Hey, why do you load the bar up with 400 pounds?"

Tom looked at me like I was nuts and replied, "Well, I would have thought that you of all people would know that in order to get stronger, I have to lift as much weight as possible every single day."

He then went on to tell me that he just knew if he kept trying to lift that weight, he'd eventually be able to do it. "You have to try and try again to succeed," he explained.

That motto might work when it comes to passing the bar exam or asking out a certain someone you've been admiring from afar, but not when you're putting heavy weights on a bar at the gym. Logic dictates that a 150-pound man like Tom should *not* be lifting 400 pounds, even if he was incorporating an advanced program into his lifestyle.

I told Tom he was lucky that he didn't land in a hospital with broken ribs or worse, and I put him on the right track with lighter weights. Today he looks like a very toned, muscular guy, and we laugh about how he used to train. However, it's not really funny—what he was doing was just plain dangerous and could have even lead to his death.

HERE'S ANOTHER QUICK STORY ABOUT MUSCLE BUILDING. I know a 25-year-old plumber named Jim who decided that he'd become a bodybuilder. Jim collected a bunch of bodybuilding magazines and decided that the "smart" way to go was to follow the program suggested by one of the sport's champions. In an almost religious way, Jim followed this man's diet and training routine down to the fine print.

After six days of this torture, Jim couldn't even lift his arms over his head, and his legs felt as if they were attached to a 2,500-pound medicine ball. He'd never been so sore in his life—in fact, just poking the guy with a finger would make him cry out in pain. Yet this was the least of his problems.

Jim's new diet had him actually doubling over in sheer agony. You see, at 165 pounds, he was eating what a 310-pound bodybuilder consumed in one day, forcing down pounds of chicken breasts, several steaks, weight-gain powder mixed with whole milk, and dozens of egg whites. This program had him consuming a whopping 700 grams of protein every 24 hours—it's no wonder that he was visiting the bathroom about ten times a day. Enough said about that.

Luckily, Jim's brother watched what he was doing and set him straight. Some people aren't as lucky because they follow a celebrity-endorsed program for months and do serious damage to their liver and kidneys, and they overtrain and rip muscles during training sessions. What you need to realize here is that programs like these work for specific individuals—no one is suggesting that it will work for everyone.

If your body goes into a revolt, stop what you're doing *immediately.* Live by this rule, because you come equipped with an alarm system that needs your attention. The scary thing is that sometimes your body gets so bogged down by a ridiculous plan that it just quits on you. Please don't become a statistic.

Brawn and Brains

When I was a teenage boy growing up in Rosedale, Queens, I was a tall, skinny type who went unnoticed by the girls and was tormented by the boys . . . until I started lifting weights. Once I saw results, I began to devour every single bodybuilding magazine and book I could get my hands on. I followed insane diet plans that would make anyone reading these pages shake their heads in disgust. There was even a short period when I ate 75 egg whites *a day* because I read in a magazine that one of my heroes did this when he was training. Later on, I learned the hard way that this was a tad excessive.

When I began to lift, there was very little information about sports nutrition. It was like walking into a fine-china store blindfolded and hoping that I didn't break anything important. When I was 14, for instance, I started to take one of those "muscle packs" you find in a health-food store, with 15 different kinds of pills in it. My great idea (and please don't ever do this) was to take three or four of these packs a day in order to become huge. One day I doubled over in pain and wound up getting my stomach pumped. I also thought that if I ate a pound of bologna, then I'd put on a pound of muscle. It's okay to laugh at this idea because even my mom rolls her eyes when I tell her this story.

Yet I'm not the only one who got it wrong. One client told me that if he just ate raw food, then he'd put a tremendous amount of muscle on. I had one word for the guy: *salmonella.* (By the way, his idea is ludicrous.) Another asked me, "If I drink five protein shakes a day mixed with whole milk and work out with weights, then will I gain more muscle? I'm converting all that extra protein into muscle." (I told him that no, this will never work, and the end result will be converting all those extra calories into fat rolls.)

My all-time favorite muscle misconception came from the woman who informed me that she only ate vegetables, which she was certain would grow her muscles at a rapid pace.

Trying not to laugh, I asked, "Why would you think this works?"

"Well, nothing grows as fast as a plant," she reasoned. "If I load up my muscles with plants, then they'll grow like a plant."

Please put down that asparagus stalk because this will never work.

Let me give you one more myth: You can gain a lean, muscular, symmetrical body without training. That's as funny to me as the lady who ate all those clumps of broccoli and then waited for her biceps to sprout.

Despite these humorous anecdotes, I hate that people look at someone who's muscular and think that they don't have a brain in their heads. First of all, it takes a fair amount of intelligence to create a great body, not to mention a strong mind. After all, Arnold Schwarzenegger became the governor of California with his charisma, acumen, *and* strength.

Having muscle is no indication of a lack of smarts. These days millions of people are trekking to the gym to work on their bodies—for example, I counsel top lawyers, doctors, scientists, and businesspeople on how to create bodies that could belong on a bodybuilding stage rather than behind a desk.

I believe that having a strong mind and strong body go together. Happy and healthy people work on both their mind and body, and it's a killer combo when both are in perfect shape.

Be Smart about the Net

Before we move on to the next chapter, I'd like to say a quick word about the Internet. The other day I was surfing the so-called health-and-fitness sites, and I couldn't believe the misinformation out there—one site actually recommended drinking six weight-gain drinks a day. I don't know if you've ever had one of these, but they contain about 900 calories. Imagine downing 5,400 extra calories a day . . . do you have any idea what a shock that would be to your body? (Not to be disgusting, but you'd also need to stock up on some Charmin because you'd be making several tours of duty in your bathroom.)

On another Website, I read that you should eat two-thirds of your daily caloric intake after you train. So if you're eating

2,500 calories a day, that means you need to eat 1,900 of them immediately after you work out. Well, you better get a bucket because you're sure to hurl if you eat that much at one time.

Obviously, you need to use your common sense when perusing the Internet, and ask your doctor before you try any diet or exercise program posted online.

CHAPTER 11

HOW BODYBUILDERS "MUSCLE UP"

A few weeks ago, I came across the old notebook in which I used to record my daily food intake during my competitive bodybuilding career. I thought you might find this to be pretty comical:

My Weekly Grocery List

- 21 pounds
- 14 pounds of chicken
- 12 pounds of fish
- 168 egg whites
- 1 big bag of potatoes
- 7 yams
- 2 giant tubs of oatmeal
- 1 20-pound bag of rice
- 2 boxes of the Original MET-Rx drink
- 8 gallons of water
- 1 big bag of broccoli
- 10 heads of lettuce, plus several cucumbers and/or tomatoes

I ate like there would be no tomorrow, and now I gasp when I look at that list. There's enough there to feed a family of five for a week! Nevertheless, I ate that mother lode without giving it a second thought. I knew that if I wanted to gain more muscle, then I needed to eat a lot of good, healthy food. Today I'm certain that my doctor would tell me that this is way too much for one person—unfortunately, it was what every bodybuilder I knew or read about was eating.

I continued to eat like that for five years, and I'm happy to report that it didn't hurt my health. Fast-forward ten years later, and I'm still alive—although I'd never recommend this type of diet to you. These days, I've discovered a healthier way to eat and grow.

THE BODYBUILDER WAY TODAY

You might not realize it, but bodybuilding has actually become the basis for many current diet plans. For example, in the best-selling book *Body-for-Life,* Bill Phillips advocates a program similar to what professional bodybuilders eat, including high amounts of protein and supplementing the diet with protein and meal replacement powders. Millions of people love this way of eating because when it's done in conjunction with the proper exercise program, it's very effective.

Years before the respected Mr. Phillips came out with his book, and even before I was born, there were bodybuilders who followed diets high in protein and low in carbs and fat, and they finished it off with protein shakes. They did so to prepare for competition because protein builds muscle and helps speed up recovery time, reduces injuries related to working out, and maintains a fit body.

It's funny that even with all the scientific advancements related to health and body issues, there are some things that never change. Bodybuilders still do basically the same thing to gain muscle, including hard training and ample supplies of protein. I've trained many pro athletes who need to carry a lot more muscle than an average person—their lives revolve around having bodies that make fans, investors, and coaches happy. These men and women also take in more than the recommended amounts of daily protein and use sports-nutrition drinks to supplement their eating plans.

I don't want anyone to go out and eat 700 grams of protein a day, but we *will* be using this nutrient to build muscle in a safer way. I suggest that you start off eating one gram per body pound if you feel comfortable with this daily eating regime. If you feel that you can handle more, then by all means, go for it. (These days I'm eating around 1.5 grams of protein per body pound because I feel that it's a good ratio for me.) The goal is to feel good—it's not about comparing numbers with someone else. You need to find out what's good for you through trial and error.

Bodybuilders do eat carbohydrates, and I'm actually an advocate of moderate amounts of them. In other words, I don't think that it's a great idea for people who want to gain muscle to stop eating carbs. Carbohydrates are your body's preferred source of energy, so when you go on a diet that restricts them, you often become lethargic. If you're trying to build muscle, then why on earth would you dismiss all the carbs? Common sense tells you that you'll be needing an infusion of energy during your workouts.

Exercise is key to building muscle or losing or gaining weight. You'll need carbohydrates to get through your time at the gym, but it must be the right ones in moderate proportions. Too many carbs will mean too many calories, and junk food won't build muscle, but will become fat. (I discussed the difference between good and bad carbs in Chapter 3.)

LIFT YOU UP

When you're trying to build muscle, you need to follow some sort of weight-resistance exercise. You won't build a substantial amount of muscle if you don't train on a regular basis, and weight training is king as far as I'm concerned. Bodybuilders know that there's nothing better than bar- and dumbbells to reach your goals.

If you're planning on building muscle, then you better plan on making the gym a part of your daily routine, much like taking a shower or brushing your teeth. I also advocate making cardiovascular exercise a part of your daily program, as it's great for stripping the body of unwanted fat and is good for your heart. (I've included a special DVD in the back of this book to get you started on your plan.)

Now you know everything that a professional bodybuilder knows. But it's time to tailor it for your own purposes . . . just turn the page.

CHAPTER 12

SPORTS-NUTRITION PRODUCTS

A long with a good diet and workout plan, athletes from the high school to pro levels have used sports-nutrition products as part of their overall fitness regimen.

Meal-replacement drinks, protein shakes, metabolic enhancers, and creatine have been used religiously by millions of people. It strikes me as strange that these products used to be looked upon negatively by those who were uneducated about them in the first place. There was even a rumor that if you downed one shake a day, it would shut down your liver. That would mean I should have been dead about 6,000 shakes ago.

Personally, I've found these items to be extremely beneficial. I've been representing MET-Rx and using their products since 1995, and I'd suggest them to anyone. If my goal was to build lean mass, then I'd implement sports-nutrition products into my overall diet and exercise program. (Remember, these aren't magic supplements—drinking or taking a pill isn't going to turn you into a hulk.) Not everyone is sold on these products as being a beneficial part of his or her personal fitness plan, and that's okay. It's your choice. I can only tell you that my personal experience with these products has been positive.

If you're going to make these products a part of your program, it's a good idea to experiment with the different brands out there and find the taste that suits you best. My brand of choice is MET-Rx, and I actually enjoy the taste of their shakes. Think about it, who wants to hold their nose when drinking a shake? So choose wisely.

My favorite thing about these drinks is the sheer convenience of them. Carrying around a MET-Rx RTD (ready to drink) is a lot easier than walking around with a chicken under my arm. I'm always running around or on an airplane, so I often don't have a kitchen at my disposal for my meals. But I can easily throw a shake into my bag.

I've met thousands of pro athletes, bodybuilders, and well-built fitness enthusiasts who have used sports-nutrition products as part of their regimen. But how and when should they be used?

DRINK SMART

I know many people who honestly believe that downing a few sports-nutrition drinks will make them muscular overnight. I'm reminded of the movie *Shrek 2,* in which the fun green guy drinks a potion that turns him into a prince. Unfortunately, there's no magical elixir that will completely transform *you,* nor is there a genie at the bottom of the protein drink who will grant you that wish of a better body. These products exist solely to supplement and assist your diet and workout plan—you'll benefit by using them in the correct manner, but they won't dramatically change your look overnight.

I have a quick story to illustrate that point. There was this great 18-year-old kid at my gym named Sam who really wanted to pack on some muscle, so he purchased some creatine and protein powder from the store and started taking it immediately. One day he saw me at the gym and asked what he should do to get bigger. I told him to take creatine and add protein shakes to his diet. Sam stopped me cold: "Frank, that's what I've been doing!" he said. "And it didn't even work."

"Well, how long have you been doing this?" I asked him.

"A whole week!" he said in a disgusted voice.

I had to remind Sam that Rome wasn't built in a day, and neither would he. In fact, we all need to stop looking for the muscle-building holy grail and realize that the process takes a lot of time.

You need to be patient and work your program. Sports-nutrition products will *only* assist your progress when used in conjunction with a proper diet and exercise program—they won't magically transform you into Sly Stallone back in the *Rocky* days. You've got to just go for it one step at a time.

MY FAVORITE MISCONCEPTION ABOUT THESE ITEMS is that you have ten seconds to live after ingesting them. I spoke earlier about how some people believe that protein shakes can cause cancer. Well, I actually had a woman come up to me on the street and tell me that the protein drink I had in my hand was going to kill me on the spot. Meanwhile, she was holding a greasy bag of fast food and looked to be about 100 pounds overweight. I'm not sure why she thought that my drink would do more damage than her cheeseburger and fries. I'll go for the shake every single time.

It also kills me when a person turns down a shake or a protein bar because they think they're too high in calories. After a yoga class, for instance, I offered my very limber instructor a protein shake, but he turned me down, saying that he didn't want to get fat.

The drink that I offered him contained 240 calories and had 40 grams of protein, 12 grams of carbohydrates, and 3 grams of fat. My instructor then reached in his bag for a granola bar, which he washed down with one of those 1,000-calorie coffee drinks. But remember that he didn't want to get fat!

I sipped my shake and didn't say another word.

SHAKES VERSUS STEROIDS

Just so we're clear, I want you to know that the sports-nutrition products I talk about in this book *have absolutely nothing to do with anabolic steroids.* I have one bit of advice about steroids: Just don't do them, since they cause numerous serious health problems. If you want a second opinion, please check with your doctor.

I can't stand when people start equating taking protein powder with injecting or ingesting steroids. The chemical breakdowns of creatine and sports-nutrition products aren't similar to steroids in any way. It's like comparing an orange with a golf club.

Steroids are illegal substances that build your muscles, including your heart, to the point of no return. There's no point in having huge, sculpted muscles when you're lying in a hospital bed hooked up to a heart monitor. That's why these substances are illegal. On the other hand, you can buy a sports-nutrition product legally anywhere in this country.

I hate when someone says, "That stuff you drink makes you all pumped up." I'd like to retort, "Of course it's just those drinks . . . it has nothing to do with the fact that I eat right and train every single day." Yeah, right.

HOW TO INCORPORATE SPORTS-NUTRITION PRODUCTS INTO YOUR DAILY ROUTINE

I believe that sports-nutrition items can be helpful when used in conjunction with a proper diet and exercise program. However, since not everyone is savvy about them, I thought I'd give you a brief description of some of the best ones on the market to help you make the right choices.

How you incorporate sports-nutrition products into your diet depends on your goals. I personally have a shake after every meal, but I also like to follow a pattern of a shake and then a meal. I've been doing this for more than ten years. Now, what kind of shake I have depends on what phase of training I'm currently involved in and what my goals are at that moment. For example, if I'm trying to gain more lean mass, I use a shake with a higher protein content.

If you're trying to gain weight, don't use a product that serves as a metabolic enhancer. The bottom line is that you must read the labels and research the ingredients in the product. (In Chapter 14, which is the Q & A, I'll answer more of your questions pertaining to specific uses of products).

There are so many products on the market that I can't describe all of them in this book. I use MET-Rx products each day and have for several years. (This doesn't mean that *you* can only use MET-Rx—it's up to you to decide what works best for your body.) I know that I like the results I've personally achieved when I combined MET-Rx with my diet and exercise program—these products work for me and my personal doc approves, so I continue to use them. Remember to check with *your* doctor before starting any fitness plan or taking any sports-nutrition product.

CHAPTER 13

THE **TRUTH** MUSCLE-BUILDING PLAN

It's finally time to begin building those muscles . . . and the first step is to lift a few fingers. Please review Chapter 3 in order to get a basic understanding of your new eating goals. The tips contained in those pages are very beneficial to your muscle building—however, we're going to adjust the food a bit here. In *this* chapter, you'll see formulas that will have you consuming more protein and slightly less fat than if you followed the exact ones for weight loss.

Building muscle requires you to eat more often and in a different manner (more protein, less fat). At the same time, you'll be following a specific workout regimen that includes weight-resistance exercises to build muscle, and cardiovascular exercises to sculpt those muscles.

Please keep in mind that you can't just do this program for a few days, quit, and then come back a week or two later if you expect real results. This is a lifestyle change that requires a commitment, but it's worth it.

Let's get started!

□—□—□

MUSCLE-BUILDING FOOD

I keep coming back to the subject of protein because this is your tool to build muscle. If you want a toned physique, you need this nutrient—but how much can you safely add to your diet? Well, if you take in the amount of protein that a professional bodybuilder eats daily, it could be harmful. I know many who eat more than three grams of protein per body pound. So if they weigh 200 pounds, they're eating at least 600 grams a day, which is an exceedingly high amount. Do not try this at home.

Personally, I stick with 1.5 grams per body pound, but your protein consumption is your choice—make the one that's healthy and feels good.

ON THE NEXT PAGE, I'VE INCLUDED THE TOP 11 FOODS that may help you increase muscle. (You can also refer to the weight-loss part of this book to remind yourself of some good versus poor food choices.) Remember that these items will only help build muscle when combined with an exercise program. *Our goal is a lifestyle change.*

THE TOP 11 FOODS THAT MAY HELP INCREASE MUSCLE MASS

1. Eggs (whites and fortified)
2. Salmon and other fish, including tuna, white fillet, cod, and orange roughy
3. Lean beef, including flank steak
4. Poultry, including chicken and turkey
5. Legumes, including pinto, kidney, and navy beans
6. Nuts, including almonds, walnuts, and cashews
7. Meal replacement powders (MRPs), ready-to-drink shakes (RTDs), and sports-nutrition bars
8. Cruciferous vegetables, including broccoli and cauliflower
9. Whole grains, including brown rice and oatmeal
10. Mollusks, including clams, oysters, and mussels
11. Yams and potatoes

SPORTS-NUTRITION PRODUCTS

Real food should be the mainstay of your program, but you should also incorporate sports-nutrition shakes and bars into your program. As I mentioned previously, I've been using these products for more than a decade—they support my protein intake, and they're a part of my everyday eating plan. These items ensure that I consume enough calories and protein each day, and they're extremely convenient.

If you're consuming MRPs, RTDs, or whey protein shakes, there are various ways you can implement them into your program. (Note that some taste better than others, so you have to experiment.) Here's a quick rundown:

1. Whey protein shakes can supplement your pro-
    tein intake. Use them with a meal, or drink them
    between meals or after a workout with some carbo-
    hydrates in the form of real food.

2. An MRP can be taken occasionally instead of a meal
    or between meals.

3. An RTD is good to drink between meals or after a
    workout.

4. *All* shakes can be taken with additional food to make
    sure that you reach your nutrient goals.

The most common and efficient way to implement shakes
into your program would look like this:

Meal 1: Food
Meal 2: A shake of your choice
Meal 3: Food
Meal 4: Shake
Meal 5: Food
Meal 6: Shake

(**Note:** Carefully read the next chapter for further specifics.)

KEEPING A MUSCLE-BUILDING JOURNAL

In the first part of this book, I advised those of you who
wanted to lose weight to keep a journal of your progress. (Please
turn to page 29 for more information.) This practice is equally
important for building mass, since recording everything you

eat will help you make the right changes to your nutritional plan. Please believe me when I tell you that muscle building is about making tweaks and adjustments as you go along. When I was competing in bodybuilding, for instance, I was constantly making changes—adding protein, subtracting carbs, and so forth.

Another good reason to keep a journal is so you can record your weight-training routines. If you're building mass, then you should be lifting heavier weights. You'll want to record all of your lifts in the journal so that you know exactly what you did and how much you lifted from workout to workout.

Let's say you bench-press 225 pounds for five reps one day and didn't record it. During your next workout, you lift 220 pounds for five reps because you forgot what you benched the previous time . . . and this is a great way to lose momentum. Five pounds can make a huge difference, trust me. Just imagine gaining five pounds a month on your bench routine—that equals a 60-pound increase over a year! It's also inspiring to look back in your records to see how far you've come with your weights.

EVERYONE IS DIFFERENT

Each month I receive thousands of letters about health and fitness. One of the recurring questions goes like this: "Why can't I build muscle like my best friend? We're both doing the identical weight and cardio workouts at the gym."

It's an age-old story: Two people join a gym at the same time and lift and eat the same, yet one person develops faster, while the other becomes depressed. The only answer I can give you is that your body is unique in how it responds to a particular nutritional plan or workout.

Don't think that your buddy has been sneaking back to the gym at three in the morning, breaking the locks, and doing an extra training session behind your back—his or her body just responds quicker. If you're a competitive type of person, it's also good to know that your friend's progress may slow, and your own will suddenly kick into high gear. Again, it's only through trial and error that you'll find the perfect nutritional muscle-building program that's personalized for your body type.

Following is a formula that you can use as a starting point. Note that high-quality protein is the center point of all the meals. That's because intense exercise increases demand for this nutrient, which supports muscle repair and growth. (Again, if you have any qualms about using this much protein, please consult your doctor before doing this plan.)

Here we go!

Starting-Point Formula for Muscle Building

1.5 grams of protein per current body weight
1 gram of carbohydrates per current body weight
.20 grams of fat x current body weight

Let's use our 200- and 125-pound friends as examples so that you can see how these particular formulas work:

Male

Current weight: 200 pounds
Daily protein intake: 200 x 1.5 = 300 grams
Daily carb intake: 200 x 1 = 200 grams
Daily fat intake: 200 x .20 = 40 grams
Total calories = 2,360

(**Note:** Carbs and protein equal four calories per gram, while fat equals nine calories per gram.)

Female

Current weight: 125 pounds

Daily protein intake: 125 x 1.5 = 187 (round off) grams

Daily carb intake: 125 x 1 = 125 grams

Daily fat intake: 125 x .20 = 25 grams

Total calories = 1,473

MEAL PLANNING

You have to make the commitment to eat at least five times a day when building muscle; in fact, some bodybuilders eat as many as *eight* meals a day. You see, if you want to *build* muscle, then you have to constantly *feed* that muscle. If you think you're going to accomplish this by only eating three meals a day, then all I have to say is good luck. I have never seen it work.

I do understand that this new eating plan will be a huge lifestyle change. You're going to have to make time every day to fit in your meals—and make them quality ones to assure that you're getting the proper nutrients to facilitate new muscle growth. That's why it's important to incorporate sports-nutrition products into your plan. They make life a lot easier for those of us with demanding schedules to get our daily nutrition in.

It's very important to plan ahead and make your meals the night before you need them. You can also carry additional protein drinks with you during the day, since they easily fit in your car or in a briefcase. Then if you can't eat a real meal for some reason, you can just down a drink and not miss a beat.

FOLLOWING ARE SOME SAMPLES THAT YOU CAN USE as a guide as you put together your own plan. Don't adhere to them religiously, because I want you to stay interested in your program. That can only happen if you put together something that suits the foods you like to eat and works best for your schedule. That is, if you're an attorney, I don't think you can be grilling your own halibut for lunch. But if you work out of your home, it's no problem. And make sure that your own individual plan satisfies your taste buds, because then you'll look forward to your meals.

Again, you don't have to be exact every single day with the grams—just get as close to your goal as possible. I understand that there will be days when you're off, so if you know that you won't be getting in all your food for the day, I suggest that you at least try to eat all of your protein.

> **FRANKLY SPEAKING:** Excuses will not help you build muscle.

Now, let's create a couple of meals based on our male and female friends from the last page:

MEAL BREAKDOWN #1
(*Male, current weight:* 200 pounds)

Each Meal

Protein: 60 grams
Carbs: 40 grams
Fat: 8 grams

SAMPLE MEAL PLANS

Meal 1

Protein: 6-egg-white omelette with 5 oz. chicken breast = 58 grams

Carbs: 1 cup oatmeal with 2 tbsp. raisins = 43 grams

Fat: 1 tbsp. peanut butter = 8 grams

Meal 2

Protein: 7 oz. turkey breast = 56 grams
Carbs: 2 slices rye bread; 2 apricots = 40 grams
Fat: .5 oz almonds = 8 grams

Meal 3

Protein: MET-Rx or any protein powder = 60 grams
Carbs: 1 cup banana and strawberries = 40 grams
Fat: .6 oz. peanuts = 8 grams

Meal 4

Protein: 7 oz. chicken breast = 56 grams

Carbs: ¾ cup steamed broccoli; 1 baked sweet potato = 37.5 grams

Fat: 1 tbsp. peanut butter = 8 grams

Meal 5

Protein: MET-Rx protein powder (or sports-nutrition product of your choice) = 60 grams

Carbohydrate: 8 oz. pineapple juice; 1 rice cake = 30 grams

Fat: .6 oz peanuts = 8 grams

(You can adjust program for 6 or 7 meals if you like.)

FRANKLY SPEAKING: In order to get to 60 grams of protein, you can use the combination of an MRP or an RTD with whey. Use protein powders with the lowest carb count, and don't forget to make adjustments to the plan when you take into consideration the carbs in sports-nutrition products. An RTD51 with a half cup of oatmeal contains 56 grams of protein. And don't worry about being exact—just get as close as you can without driving yourself insane.

MEAL BREAKDOWN #2
(Female, current weight: 125 pounds)

Each Meal

Protein: 37 grams
Carbs: 25 grams
Fat: 5 grams

SAMPLE MEAL PLANS

Meal 1

Protein: MET-Rx or any other protein powder = 37 grams
Carbs: 1 cup oatmeal = 25 grams
Fat: ½ tbsp. peanut butter = 4 grams

Meal 2

Protein: 4 oz. turkey breast = 32 grams
Carbs: 2 slices rye bread = 32 grams
Fat: .33 oz. peanuts = 4 grams

Meal 3

Protein: 4.5 oz. chicken breast = 36 grams
Carbs: ½ cup rice = 25 grams
Fat: .25 oz. cashews = 3.5 grams

Meal 4

Protein: MET-Rx or any other protein = 37 grams
Carbs: 1 cup oatmeal = 27 grams
Fat: ½ tbsp. peanut butter = 4 grams

Meal 5

Protein: 5 oz. halibut = 36 grams

Carbs: 1 cup lettuce and 1 cup broccoli with 2 tbsp. fat-free dressing = 30 grams

Fat: 1 oz. olives = 8 grams

TIME TO PICK <u>YOUR</u> MEALS

Variety is the key to sticking to your plan, so please use the Master Food List at the back of the book (see page 157) to pick different foods to implement into your program.

Also keep in mind that it's going to be very difficult to cook five or six meals a day, seven days a week—you need a little convenience in your life, which is where sports-nutrition products come in. My advice is to find one you like because you'll be using it on a daily basis. Go down to your local nutrition store, buy a couple of the drinks, and perform your own personal taste test. When you find one that you enjoy, check out the other flavors made by that particular brand. I'm sure that you'll find some you love and some you hate, but keep trying until you zero in on one or two that are acceptable.

ADJUSTING YOUR PLAN

Remember that this plan is a starting point—you'll have to tweak it as you go along, while also keeping a close eye on how your body reacts to the plan. Give yourself a two-week period so that your body can adjust to the diet, and then make the necessary corrections.

If you find that you can't handle the allotted amount of protein, then scale it back. If you feel as if you need more carbs because you lack energy, then please add some in. Your workout program (which takes into consideration your body's recovery and the intensity of your exercise) will dictate many of the changes you make to your nutritional program. The goal is to keep progressing in a positive manner.

CHEAT MEALS

Just as with my weight-loss plan, you're entitled to a cheat meal after two weeks of sticking to the program. After that period of time, you can have one cheat meal every week. So enjoy that pizza, but just make sure that you go right back on your plan after the last bite. Oh, and please don't miss any workouts because you're stuck in the pizzeria extending that one meal to two more. Use some discretion when it comes to the size of your cheat meal.

FRANKLY SPEAKING: Eating for three hours at a buffet isn't a cheat meal—it's a gorge session.

Working Out

A quick heads-up: If you plan on building a muscular body, then you better do some sort of weight-resistance and cardiovascular exercise. The weight training is for building your muscles, while the cardio is for sculpting them.

If you just follow my nutritional plan and don't exercise, then the only thing that you'll be gaining is fat. Be sure to check out the DVD that comes with this book for a great routine. (And for more intense muscle-building workouts, look into Level 5 and the expert exercise techniques in my book *The TRUTH*.)

Overtraining

I've already made it pretty clear that the key to losing body fat and maintaining a healthy body is a great diet and regular exercise. But how much is too much?

Well, just like anything else, too much of a good thing isn't good for *you.* I know many people who get addicted to exercise in the same way they used to be chocolate-chip-cookie junkies. I know that your body feels great after each workout, so it's natural to think, *Hey, I don't want to do this four days a week—I'll do it <u>seven</u> days a week. No, wait, I'll exercise twice a day, seven days a week.* This is called overtraining, and this can be just as bad as not exercising at all.

How do you know if you're guilty of this practice? Well, be honest when you look at some of the symptoms that I list next. If any of them pertain to you, please turn down the intensity a notch, sit out a day, or slow down. You body will thank you.

SIGNS OF OVERTRAINING:

1. Loss of appetite. Overtraining can cause an increase in hormones such as epinephrine and norepinephrine, which can inhibit appetite.

2. Excessive fatigue. If you never give your body the proper rest, it will never recuperate—you'll keep tearing your muscles down without giving them a chance to rebuild, although they're desperate to do so. You're working too hard, so put on the brakes.

3. Normal workouts become harder. If workouts that you used to do with no problem are becoming extremely demanding and strenuous, it's a sign of overtraining. Lack of proper rest will force your body to underperform, even during the most basic workout. If you could do 30 minutes on the treadmill with no problem two weeks ago, and now you can barely get through 15 without feeling like you're going to need a nap, then guess what? Your body needs a rest!

4. Muscle soreness and joint pain. If you keep working out over and over without proper rest, then your muscles and joints will break down and begin to ache. Don't ignore these signs, because they can lead to a serious injury.

5. Increased illness—especially of the respiratory nature. When your body is overworked, your immune system breaks down, leaving you more susceptible to colds. If you keep getting sick, it might not be from the kid in your morning car pool. Ease up a bit on the working out and see what happens.

I want you to work out at your own fitness level while flexing your common sense, too. I know that it's easy to get so "into" a new fitness program that you want to see maximum results at the quickest rate possible. The truth is that you can't reverse ten years of sitting on the couch while lifting Doritos to your mouth in the span of two weeks. If only . . .

I like the saying "Slow but steady wins the race," which really does apply to losing, gaining, or building muscles. It takes consistency, determination, and a good plan to achieve your fitness goals. In other words, you don't need an insane workout schedule, but a smart one. I'm afraid that more is just not better here . . . after all, exercise is not like money or vacations.

I know how hard it is to pull back at the gym when your enthusiasm gets the better of you, but you have to get your mind-set under control if you want to really get in good, life-long shape. *Too much exercise will not make you achieve results any faster; in fact, it could actually have the opposite effect.* People who excessively exercise are risking more than poor performance—they're risking their health.

For more questions or concerns you may have on muscle building, please turn the page.

CHAPTER 14

MUSCLE-BUILDING Q & A

This chapter contains some of the questions I'm routinely asked about muscle building and sports-nutrition products. I hope that my answers will help you clear up any confusion, too.

Question: "Should I drink my shakes (whey, MRPs, or RTDs) on days that I don't train with weights?"

Frank says: You should absolutely drink them, even on the days you miss a training session. You see, your muscles need protein and nutrients *all the time,* not just on the days you lift. In order to gain muscle, you need to give your body the proper rest and recuperation it needs. On those off days, your body will still need the additional protein and nutrients. (Also, make sure that you don't lower your protein intake from your food plan to compensate.)

Question: "Should I eat immediately after I work out?"

Frank says: Yes, you need food, but you should start with water to replenish fluid loss. You have a one-hour window to eat after you train—this is when your muscles will absorb the most nutrients and glycogen (an energy reserve) will be replaced most efficiently.

Question: "Should I eat before I train?"

Frank says: If you're trying to burn body fat, then the best time to do so is first thing in the morning on an empty stomach. This is when your glycogen stores are at their lowest, so you'll burn stored body fat. If you want to get the most out of your cardio performance, then you should eat lightly about one hour before you exercise (fruit or low-starch vegetables such as carrots and green beans will do the trick). The hour will allow time for digestion and still give you the energy bump you need to do your cardio.

Your other option is to eat a larger meal—consisting of protein, healthy fats, and carbohydrates—two or three hours before working out. If you lack energy, then you can use one of the many energy drinks out there. I've personally used Worldwide Sports Nutrition Super Charged Tea before working out. But there are also drinks on the market that were developed to promote nitric oxide synthesis, and carbohydrate drinks are readily available for you to sustain energy during workouts. I suggest that you do your research on all of these products and choose one that's specific to your personal needs and goals.

One final note here: Do be sure that you know what ingredients you're ingesting. Many people have heart conditions, for instance, so drinking a beverage that contains excessive amounts of caffeine is a recipe for disaster. I want you to be smart and check labels—and if you don't understand an ingredient, please check it out with your doctor.

Question: "What kind of sports drink should I use after my workout: a carbohydrate or protein drink?"

Frank says: Athletes need carbs and fluids to replace glycogen and water loss during exercise, but protein is also important to repair and build the muscle tissue. So, to answer your question, you should take in a sports drink that contains both.

I grab a carbohydrate drink and a whey protein shake after I work out, but you can also mix your protein shake with some fruit to get both carbs and protein. Just be sure that you stay away from high-fat, high-calorie weight gainers. (You could also eat a bar that contains protein and carbs.)

Question: "Is a protein shake a good substitute for a meal?"

Frank says: A meal should consist of protein, carbohydrates, and fat. Now, since a protein shake mainly consists of protein with trace amounts of carbohydrates and fat, this will *not* replace a meal. Instead, a shake should be used to supplement your overall protein intake. I know many bodybuilders who have used an MRP as a substitute for a meal . . . but not every meal.

The majority of your daily calories should be from regular food. I always make sure that I'm eating at least three meals a day of solid sustenance, and I'd never replace one of them with a shake. I always do a meal (solid food) and then a shake, or vice versa.

Question: "I've heard that too much protein is dangerous. Is this true or false?"

Frank says: There's been quite a bit of recent research done on this subject because of the increased number of popular high-protein programs out there, such as the Atkins and South Beach diets. Some findings have suggested that too much protein can leave you dehydrated and increase your risk of kidney stones as well as some forms of cancer. On the other hand, too much carbohydrate and fat consumption has been proven to be associated with numerous health risks such as heart disease.

On the positive side, there have been studies done in France that appeared in the *American Journal of Physiology,* which revealed that a high-protein diet helped a group of rats maintain a lower body weight (18 percent lower, to be exact) than the control group, even while feeding freely on high-protein foods. High-protein intake also resulted in healthy liver and kidney functions, outstanding blood chemistry, healthier blood-sugar regulation, and improved glucose tolerance in the rodents. No negative effects were found from a high-protein diet—all of the rats subjected to it weighed less than when they started, and their organs showed no signs of abnormal functions. However, the study was done on rats, not humans.

The bottom line is that it's up to you if you want to take more than the recommended amount of daily protein. I've made the choice to eat between one to two grams of protein per body pound, and I think that the 600 to 800 grams that some bodybuilders take in is way too much. Your body can't process all that protein into amino acids, and much of it will be excreted as waste—meaning that your kidneys and liver will be doing a lot of work to get the excess protein out of your body. While this might not cause any short-term problems, you don't want to overwork your organs over the course of several years. I believe that too much of anything is never good, but again it's up to you and your doctor.

Question: "What's the maximum number of shakes I should drink in one day?"

Frank says: First, let me say that you should never replace all of your meals with shakes. No matter how good they are for you, they're not substitutes for food. Having said that, I know people who drink four shakes a day and have no problem whatsoever, yet there are others who can't handle more than two. It depends on the shakes, your body weight, and your fitness goals. I have three MET-Rx RTD shakes a day, and sometimes I drink a MET-Rx Whey shake as well. Again, it's your personal choice.

Question: "What is the difference between an RTD, MRP, and whey protein?"

Frank says: The simple answer is that each has a different nutritional breakdown. Whey protein is a protein supplement used to enhance the amount of protein you're currently taking in—the drinks are very low in carbohydrates and have to be mixed. Just as its name implies, RTDs are premixed and ready to drink. The breakdown of an RTD depends on what kind you purchase—they can range from 18 to 60 grams of protein, with the carb count varying depending on the product. MRPs have to be mixed, and their nutritional breakdown also varies.

Question: "Is it true that protein bars aren't that good for you?"

Frank says: It depends on the nutritional breakdown of the bar. It helps to become label savvy—if a specific bar reads that it's too high in trans fats and sugar, then you should take a pass, because it will hurt your program. Anyone who's pursuing a high-protein diet or is a fitness enthusiast will require more protein than the average person, and a bar can help fulfill that need. There are also bars that are made specifically for endurance and are used by athletes because they have a high carbohydrate content. I enjoy MET-Rx Protein Plus bars because they have about 32 grams of protein, 32 carbohydrates, and 0 grams of trans fat. They're also enriched with 21 vitamins and minerals and have no added sucrose or fructose. This sounds a lot healthier to me than a greasy cheeseburger and fries from the drive-through.

Question: "I don't want to be a bodybuilder, but I'd like to have more lean muscle mass. Should I still use protein bars and shakes?"

Frank says: Whether or not you want to become a bodybuilder is irrelevant. There are millions of people in the gym who train to be fit and healthy, and the majority of them make sports-nutrition products part of their daily regimen. Some people choose not to use sports-nutrition products and also make gains. I personally believe that when shakes and bars are used in conjunction with a proper diet and exercise program, they are helpful. It's your choice.

Question: "What exactly is creatine?"

Frank says: Creatine is a naturally occurring amino acid (protein building block) found mainly in muscles. You see, 50 percent of the amino acids in our bodies are ingested through the foods we eat, while the other 50 percent is made in the liver, kidney, and pancreas—roughly one-third of this amount is found in its free form as creatine, while the remainder is bound to phosphate and called *creatine phosphate* or *phosphocreatine.* Studies conducted in both animals and people have shown that creatine supplements improve strength and lean muscle mass during high-intensity, short-duration exercise (such as weight lifting). Again, it's up to you. Do your own research. I would do my own research before putting anything in my body.

Question: "Isn't creatine dangerous?"

Frank says: I've known dozens of people who have used it with great results and no adverse effects. Creatine sales have been in the millions for years—I'd hope that if it were a danger to our health, then it wouldn't be made available to the general public. I can only give you my personal experiences with the product, and they've all been positive.

However, there have been individuals who have reported adverse effects, so if you have any concerns, then you should definitely seek the advice of a health-care professional to help you decide.

Question: "What's glutamine, and can it help build muscle?"

Frank says: Glutamine is the most common amino acid found in your muscles, and it's needed throughout your body for optimal performance. It has a long list of benefits for the body that would fill the rest of this book. In short, glutamine is the most important component of muscle protein. So, yes, there are studies that show it can aid you in the muscle-building process.

Question: "What's the difference between Metamyosyn protein and whey?"

Frank says: Whey protein is only one type of protein, while Metamyosyn is a mix of high-quality milk proteins, casein, and whey proteins. The Metamyosyn protein was developed by a physician, based on metabolic research on supporting lean muscle mass.

There are numerous types of whey protein, including whey protein concentrate, whey protein isolate, and hydrolyzed whey protein. Whey protein is a pure, natural, high-quality protein from cow's milk—and in its purest form (whey protein isolate), it contains very little fat, cholesterol, or lactose.

Question: "Are amino acids important for building muscle?"

Frank says: Amino acids are found in meat, poultry, eggs, fish, dairy products, and (of course) select bars and shakes. Are they important for building muscle? Let me put it this way: Are tires important to a car?

Amino acids are the building blocks of protein. You need 20 amino acids to build the various proteins used in the repair, growth, and maintenance of body tissues. You don't have to work that hard for the first 11 of those amino acids because your body makes them as a courtesy. But the other nine, which are called essential amino acids, come from your diet. So don't let your body down here!

APPENDIX

TRAINING 101

There's a little something extra included in this book that I think will help your training a great deal. I've added a special-edition workout DVD that will be like having me in your home, acting as your personal trainer.

But before you pop in the disc and start working up a sweat, I thought that I should give you some final information on cardio and weight training.

Much of the material in this Appendix comes from my first two books. Now you may be wondering why I didn't just concoct something new for the market—and the answer is that I'm someone who stands true to what I believe about training. You won't find me flip-flopping and reinventing the wheel just so I can be trendy. My opinions about nutrition and exercise haven't changed since I wrote my first book three years ago.

In *this* book, I've stressed how important it is to incorporate both cardiovascular and weight-training exercises into your life. I realize that it's going to take a major change for you to make an exercise program a daily part of your life, but to borrow a line from the Nike company: "Just do it."

I'll talk a bit more about cardio in the next section, but right now I'd like to focus on weight training. I believe there's no better workout than one that includes weights.

THE HEALTH BENEFITS OF WEIGHT TRAINING

— **You'll reduce the risk of heart disease.** Studies have shown that weight training can indeed improve cardiovascular health in many ways. It can help decrease LDL (or "bad") cholesterol, increase HDL (or "good" cholesterol), and lower blood pressure. If you mix in some cardio with your weight training, then you can maximize these benefits.

— **You'll reduce the risk of diabetes.** Certain studies have shown that weight-resistance exercise can increase glucose utilization in the body and improve the way the body processes sugar, which may lower your risk of diabetes.

— **You'll reduce the risk of osteoporosis.** Weigh training has been proven to increase spinal bone mineral density by a substantial percentage. Women of all ages are trekking off to the gym these days and pumping iron for the first time in their lives because they want to keep their bones strong. The combination of dietary calcium and lifting weights has been called "the one-two punch" against osteoporosis.

— **You may improve your mental health.** It isn't all about *physical* health when it comes to weight training—you'll also increase your self-esteem because you'll feel more empowered after training. You'll gain more confidence because you're stronger and you look better.

— **Wait . . . there's more!** Weight training will obviously make you stronger, which will help prevent injury. Not only will your muscles get stronger, but so will your connective tissues, which will help increase your body's joint stability. How many millions of Americans suffer from lower-back pain? Weight training in conjunction with a good nutritional plan can help alleviate or eliminate that discomfort.

— **And then there's my personal favorite reason to lift weights.** No, it's not so that I look great in short-sleeved shirts. The best reason to pump iron is because we're getting smarter as a nation about exercise. Most of us know that when we cut calories and don't exercise, we'll lose muscle as well as fat. When we lose muscle, our bodies become less efficient at burning fat, and when we gain muscle, our bodies burn fat more efficiently.

If your goal is weight loss or even weight gain, you don't want to put on fat. So, what are you waiting for? Get a dumbbell in each hand—after all, it turns that out there's nothing dumb about them.

BONUS WEIGHT-LIFTING Q & A

Question: "How do I pick the right weight to lift?"

Frank says: The only way you're going to answer this question is by trial and error. This means that you should experiment: Start out by picking up a light weight, see if you can do a set, and move on from there. If you start curling and find that you can do 100 reps, it's not because you've suddenly developed superhuman strength. You're working out with weights that are too light, so you're not going to see many results. Don't get irritated during this trial period because it takes time to find the right weight for you.

Question: "How do I know when to increase the weight?"

Frank says: If your workout program indicates that you're supposed to do ten reps and you get to that number easily, then it's a surefire eureka moment at the gym (or in your living room). But don't throw a party . . . just add some weight to your workout. And congratulations—you're getting stronger!

I want you to be honest with yourself on this subject—because if a weight is too light and you continue to take the easy way out, then you're not building strength or causing enough overload to build muscles. This isn't rocket science, so please don't let a trainer at a gym convince you that it's a difficult process. Just pay attention to how tough it is to lift the weight, and then gradually adjust as necessary.

Question: "How long should I rest between sets?"

Frank says: This is based on your own personal fitness level. I strongly suggest that if you're just starting out, then it helps to rest for 90 seconds between sets or until your normal breathing returns.

Question: "Should I warm up before I train?"

Frank says: Yes, you should definitely warm up to make sure that your muscles are ready to go before you start weight training. I like to loosen up by doing a five-minute walk on the treadmill followed by a full-body stretching routine. This is a great way to mentally and physically prepare for a weight-training session.

A FINAL WORD ON CARDIO AND CALORIE BURNING

As I've said may times in these pages, cardio helps burn body fat. But believe me, I know that it's the most hated form of exercise. The treadmill and the StairMaster get more dirty looks than most machines at the gym, and my own clients will come up with any excuse not to endure their 30- to 45-minute sessions.

I hate to break it to you, but cardiovascular exercise is crucial to the success of your program, especially if you want to lose weight. Don't shoot the messenger!

WHY YOU NEED TO STOP MAKING EXCUSES AND START DOING CARDIO

- It increases your energy for sex and lung capacity for living. (I thought I'd mention sex first to get your attention!)

- It reduces the risk of heart attack.

- It helps lower your blood pressure.

- It naturally boosts your metabolism.

- It alleviates stress.

Now aren't those good reasons to make cardio a regular, every-day thing?

THE WINNING COMBO OF CARDIO AND WEIGHT TRAINING

Go to any gym and you'll encounter people who swear that you don't need to weight-train if you do cardio, while another group will avow that you don't have to do cardio if you weight-train. Both are completely wrong.

The most effective way to permanently lose weight is to combine cardio, strength training, and a healthy diet. If you're trying to achieve a trim midsection, then you've got to lose body fat and not just drop weight. Cardio will help you do so by burning excess calories, which will reduce your body fat (if you're also following the right eating program, that is).

WHEN SHOULD YOU DO IT?

If your only form of cardio lately has been walking to the doughnut shop around the block, then I'd say that *any* time you make to do cardio is the right time.

For the rest of you, the best time to do cardio (or fat burning) is first thing in the morning on an empty stomach. That doesn't mean you should have a glass of orange juice or a shake and then do your cardio because liquids don't count. (See, I've heard all of the excuses in the world.) An empty stomach means *totally empty.* This is the perfect time for cardio because you haven't eaten in six to eight hours, and your body will search for some carbs to burn when you start to work out. But your body will be out of luck because your stomach is empty—so it will have no other choice but to go after your stored body fat.

If you choose to do cardio later in the day after a few meals, all you'll be burning off are the calories you've just eaten. This is better than nothing, but ultimately I want you to achieve maximum results from your workout.

Many clients ask me if they should do their cardio before or after they train with weights. There have been numerous studies on this topic with conflicting answers. My personal preference is to do my weight training before I do my cardio. This practice results in my body burning up fat as an energy source because I've already depleted my glycogen levels with the weight-training workout. (Cardio can also help with the removal of lactic acid, which builds up after weight training.)

A FEW WORDS TO THE WISE BEFORE YOU START

I strongly recommend that you purchase a heart-rate monitor (HRM). It will make your workout much more effective and safe, since you'll get the most out of every training session. It's like having your very own personal trainer who tells you when to slow down or speed up.

If you want to reach your fitness goals, then you have to train in the correct zone. An HRM is the most accurate way to continually measure your heart rate and ensure that you're working out at the right intensity level. Besides being crucial to your performance, this handy device will let you know if you're overdoing it or when you've recovered properly during interval training.

WHAT'S AN "RHR"?

RHR stands for *resting heart rate,* or the number of times your heart beats per minute when your body is at rest. By knowing your RHR, you can gauge your workouts more efficiently and measure your improvements more precisely.

You can determine your resting heart rate very easily. Simply relax and then place your two fingers on the side of your neck to find your pulse. Next, count the number of beats you feel in one minute. The average RHR for a man is 70 beats per minute (bpm), while for women it's 75 bpm. Athletes will have a lower RHR because it takes less effort and fewer bpm for their hearts to pump blood through their bodies.

WHAT'S AN "MHR"?

MHR stands for *maximum heart rate* or the top number of beats your heart pumps in a minute. When you do cardio, it's important to do it at the right level.

I know that you're probably wondering what the right level is, and this is where heart-rate zone training comes in. By adhering to the simple formula that follows, you can find the correct zone to train in:

MHR for women = 226 - your age
MHR for men = 220 - your age
Example: For a 25-year-old man, the equation would be 220 - 25 = 195.

WHAT'S A "THR"?

THR stands for *target heart rate*, and the equation to figure it out is: MHR x .55 (55%) to MHR x .90 (90%). So, based on the 25-year-old above, it would be from 195 x .55 to 195 x .90. That means that this guy's target rate would be between 107.25 and 175.5 bpm.

If you're not so great at math and can't figure out this equation, here's a chart that illustrates the right MHR broken down by age groups:

AGE	50% MHR	60% MHR	70% MHR	80% MHR
18–25	99	119	139	159
26–30	95	119	139	153
31–36	93	112	130	149
37–42	90	108	126	144
42–50	86	103	121	138
51–58	83	99	116	133
59–65	79	95	110	126
65+	76	91	106	121

FRANKLY SPEAKING: I'd like you to always wear an HRM during cardiovascular exercise so that you can monitor your heart rate at all times.

WHAT RANGE SHOULD YOU TRAIN IN?

The range you should be training in depends upon your level of fitness. If you're a beginner, you should stay within 55–60% of your MHR; but if your goal is to lose body fat, then you need to be within 60–70% of your MHR. (This is also known as the "weight-management zone.") Working out at 70–80% of your MHR will help improve function of your lungs, heart, and respiratory rate. Working out at 80–90% will further help endurance and increase speed, but shouldn't be done without supervision.

Exercising at 90% of your MHR is the anaerobic range, which should only be done in short bursts. This range is so intense that your cardiovascular system can't get oxygen to the muscles, yet it's commonly used in interval training routines to help performance. (Be very careful if you train in this range because you can easily get hurt.)

How Much and How Long Should You Do It?

The degree and duration to which you do cardio all depends upon your level of fitness. If you're a beginner, no one expects you to swim the English Channel or hike up Mount Everest. If the only cardio you've done recently is in your mind while you watched TV, then too bad cardio doesn't work through osmosis, huh?

On a serious note, if you really haven't exercised in the last year, then the first thing you should do is make an appointment for a physical. Once you get the medical A-OK that you're fit enough to start, then you need to go slowly, and gradually build up during your sessions.

I'd suggest that beginners start by simply walking for 15 minutes three days a week. (Try to keep your MHR at 60%.) After a week or so, if you feel as though you're ready to move on and the sessions are becoming easier, then add five minutes to each one. If you do so consistently, you'll be amazed at how fast you start moving. The goal is to make cardio a daily part of your life and not a temporary fix, so it's fine to start with less time and build up. It's much worse to do 45 minutes, exhaust yourself, and then not do it again for two months because it's just too defeating.

If you're not a beginner, then there's no definite plan to follow—each person reacts differently to the amount and frequency of the cardio they do. For general fitness, you should exercise between three to five times a week for 20 to 30 minutes. For fat burning, alternating between high- and low-intensity cardio four to six days a week for 20- to 60-minute sessions is best.

Obviously, you'll only do the high-intensity cardio for a lesser time (such as 20 minutes). Keep in mind that cardio works in conjunction with your diet program, so if you're eating 500 more calories a day than you're burning, you're still going to gain weight . . . no matter how much time you log on the treadmill. Also, those extra 500 calories a day will add up to 3,500 calories by the end of the week, and that translates into a one-pound gain. For all of you who tell me that you work out like demons but never lose weight, this is probably the problem.

> **FRANKLY SPEAKING:** If you're trying to gain weight, don't exclude cardio. Just make sure that you're eating enough—and remember that I want you to gain lean muscle mass.

SAMPLE PROGRAM

On the next page is a schedule that appears in my book *The TRUTH,* and I thought you'd benefit from seeing how a cardio plan can look:

LEVEL 2 CARDIO PROGRAM

WEEK 1	WEEK 2	WEEK 3	WEEK 4 (and beyond)
Monday: 30 minutes biking or walking at 50–70% MHR	**Monday:** 35 minutes biking or walking at 50–70% MHR	**Monday:** 40 minutes biking or walking at 50–70% MHR	**Monday:** 40 minutes biking or walking at 50–70% MHR
Wednesday: 30 minutes biking or walking at 50–70% MHR	**Wednesday:** 35 minutes biking or walking at 50–70% MHR	**Wednesday:** 40 minutes biking or walking at 50–70% MHR	**Wednesday:** 40 minutes biking or walking at 50–70% MHR
Friday: 30 minutes biking or walking at 50–70% MHR	**Friday:** 35 minutes biking or walking at 50–70% MHR	**Friday:** 40 minutes biking or walking at 50–70% MHR	**Friday:** REST—you deserve it
Weekend: Fun physical activity—Rollerblading, playing with a pet, etc.	**Weekend:** Golf, tennis, swimming, or any other fun physical activity	**Weekend:** Shopping, sightseeing, or other fun physical activity	**Weekend:** Yoga, kickboxing, etc.

FRANKLY SPEAKING: You should never just stop doing cardio abruptly. Add a cooldown to your workout to bring yourself down gradually and decrease the intensity. If you're running on the treadmill at 7.0, for instance, don't just stop and jump off. You should decrease the speed and gradually slow down until your heart rate comes back down to normal. Your body will thank you for it.

Following is a chart from *Frank Sepe's ABS-olutely Perfect Plan for a Flatter Stomach,* which helpfully illustrates how many calories certain cardio activities burn in ten minutes:

ACTIVITY AND CALORIES/ 10 MINS.	123-LB. WOMAN	170-LB. MAN
Basketball	77	106
Cycling (5.5 mph)	36	49
Cycling (9.4 mph)	56	74
Cycling (racing)	95	130
Dance exercise (high-impact aerobics)	94	124
Dance exercise (low-impact aerobics)	80	105
Football	74	102
Racquetball	76	107
Rope skipping (slow)	82	116
Rope skipping (fast)	100	142
Running (8 mins./mile)	113	150
Running (11½ mins./mile)	76	100
Skiing (cross country)	80	106
Soccer	78	107
StairMaster	88	122
Step aerobics (4-inch bench)	48	66
Step aerobics (6-inch bench)	58	80
Step aerobics (8-inch bench)	67	92
Step aerobics (10-inch bench)	75	104
Swimming (backstroke)	95	130
Swimming (breaststroke)	91	125
Swimming (fast crawl)	87	120
Swimming (slow crawl)	95	130
Swimming (sidestroke)	68	90
Swimming (treading water)	35	48
Tennis (singles)	61	81
Volleyball	28	39
Weight training (super circuit)	104	137
Weight training (muscular strength)	44	60
Weight training (muscular endurance)	58	80
Walking (3.5 mph)	45	59

(Data for this table was taken from *Reebok Instructor News,* Volume 5, Number 2, 1997.)

THE MET-RX/FRANK SEPE DVD

You're finally ready to enjoy the DVD that comes with this book. After reading my words for the past couple hundred pages, please feel free to yell back at me during a tough part of the workout!

You'll find two different weight-training programs on the disc. The first is a beginner routine that you can do either at home or in the gym. The only equipment you need is a pair of adjustable dumbbells and a utility bench.

For those of you who think you need to run out and buy a gym membership, let me remind you again that you can easily work out in the privacy of your own home. I have a few clients who have never been to a gym before, and they feel intimidated walking into the weight room with all the muscle guys. That's a valid concern, although I've seen men and women of all ages and fitness levels pumping iron.

If you do feel a bit shy about working out publicly, just use the beginner program on the DVD as a starting point at home, and then maybe you'll want to look into gyms eventually. There are many people who believe that you have to join the most expensive fitness center in town or hire a top personal trainer in order to succeed at keeping in shape. Well, just know that I trained in my basement for four years before I even signed up to join a commercial gym. I made some fantastic strides in that basement.

Training at home also makes sense because you might be one of those people who has no time to get to a workout center because of your job, your kids, or your mate. Why not bring the gym to you—and a 24-hour, seven-day-a-week gym at that, which is complete with your own clean shower? You can watch your DVD and learn the exercises at home with me right there on your screen.

THE DIFFERENT WORKOUTS

On the DVD, I'll walk you through every exercise from start to finish while demonstrating how each one is correctly done. As I mentioned, there are two different workouts on the disc:

1. The beginner program is a three-day-a-week, full-body plan. It's perfect for the person who has a busy, hectic lifestyle and likes to kick back on the weekends. And, as I already mentioned, the only equipment you'll need is a bench and some dumbbells. It couldn't be easier unless I came over and did it for you! (Sorry, I can't be in every living room at all hours—my wife likes me at home.)

2. The intermediate program is a three-day-on, two-day-off workout, which means that you'll be training for three days in a row and then taking two days off. This routine incorporates both free weights and machines . . . so you must leave the living room. (Yes, this routine requires a gym.)

The DVD will walk you through each exercise from start to finish while I demonstrate exactly how to do each exercise. I'll also offer helpful tips while doing the reps.

ONE MORE THING ABOUT YOUR DVD

Along with the two workout programs, the disc also includes some basic nutritional information, along with a few comments about MET-Rx products because they're the brand that I personally use.

The DVD is intended to increase your level of physical fitness. The instructions and advice contained within are not in any way intended to be a substitute for counseling from your health-care professional, whom you should always consult before beginning this or any other diet, support, exercise, or fitness program.

Now pop in the DVD and enjoy the show!

MY PERSONAL PLAN

The number one question people ask me when they see me is simple: "Are you really leaving that parking spot?" Just kidding. Since I'm constantly asked what I do on a daily basis to maintain my body, I thought I'd share my answer with you here. (Please keep in mind that these plans were developed for my personal body type and goals, and I don't recommend your trying this exact regimen. However, if you'd like to explore training on a deeper level, then please check out my first two books, *The TRUTH* and *Frank Sepe's ABS-olutely Perfect Plan for a Flatter Stomach.*)

Remember that you can't change your body overnight—it takes time and commitment to make lasting changes, but it is so worth it. There's nothing better than looking and feeling great, so make the choice to change your life. Do it today . . . and for the rest of your life.

And put down that muffin!

MY BODYBUILDING DIET, OFF-SEASON

Meal 1: 12 egg whites, turkey sausage, 6 banana pancakes

Meal 2: The Original MET-Rx drink mix, tuna on whole wheat

Meal 3: 16 oz. beef, pasta, vegetables

Meal 4: The Original MET-Rx drink mix, bowl of rice

Meal 5: 16 oz. turkey, pasta, vegetables

Meal 6: MET-Rx shake, bowl of rice

Meal 7: Whatever I want

ALTERNATE OFF-SEASON BODYBUILDING DIET

Meal 1: 6 egg whites, 6 oz. turkey, 1 cup of oatmeal, 1 tsp. peanut butter

Meal 2: The Original MET-Rx drink mix (mixed with skim milk), 2 bananas

Meal 3: 16 oz. salmon, pasta, vegetables

Meal 4: The Original MET-Rx drink mix (mixed with ½ cup yogurt), some peanut butter

Meal 5: 12 oz. turkey, shrimp, pasta, vegetables

Meal 6: The Original MET-Rx drink mix, 1 peanut-butter sandwich

Meal 7: Whatever I want

BODYBUILDING PLAN, PRE-CONTEST

Meal 1: 12 egg whites, ½ cup oatmeal (dry)

Meal 2: The Original MET-Rx drink mix (mixed with water)

Meal 3: Chicken, baked potato, vegetables, green salad (topped with olive oil)

Meal 4: The Original MET-Rx drink mix (mixed with water)

Meal 5: Orange roughy, 1 small yam, green salad (topped with olive oil)

Meal 6: MET-Rx original drink mix

My Modeling Maintenance Diet

Meal 1: 12 egg whites, turkey sausage, oatmeal

Meal 2: The Original MET-Rx drink mix (mixed with water)

Meal 3: Turkey, yam, vegetables, green salad

Meal 4: MET-Rx RTD 51 Cookies & Cream or MET-Rx Protein Plus

Meal 5: Chicken, brown rice, vegetables, salad (topped with olive oil)

THE **TRUTH** MASTER FOOD LIST

Finally, I ask that you never underestimate the importance of eating correctly. It can spell the difference between success and failure, so be sure to follow the programs I've outlined in this book as closely as possible. Combine the right level of healthy eating with your workout plan, and you'll be on your way to greater health; higher self-esteem; and a lean, hard, and sexy body.

Enjoy! And drop me a line to let me know how you're progressing.

PROTEIN SOURCES		
Food	**Serving Size**	**Protein**
MEAT/EGGS		
Beef, flank steak	1 oz. raw weight	7 (3 fat)
Beef, ground	1 oz. raw weight	7 (5 fat)
Beef, top round, eye of round or full round (lean only)	1 oz. raw weight	9
Chicken breast, boneless	1 oz. cooked weight	8
Cottage cheese, fat-free	½ cup	7
Egg substitute	¼ cup	6
Egg white	1 large	3
Protein powder, such as MET-Rx Protein Plus	1 scoop	16
Turkey breast, boneless	1 oz. cooked weight	8
Veal (lean only) braised or stewed	1 oz. cooked weight	10
FISH/SEAFOOD		
Bass	1 oz. cooked weight	7 (1 fat)
Clams	1 oz. cooked weight (meat only)	7 (1 fat)
Cod	1 oz. cooked weight	6
Crab	1 oz. cooked weight (meat only)	6
Haddock	1 oz. cooked weight	7
Halibut	1 oz. cooked weight	7
Lobster	1 oz. cooked weight (meat only)	6
Orange roughy	1 oz. cooked weight	5
Salmon	1 oz. cooked weight	6 (3 fat)
Scallops	1 oz. raw weight	5
Sea bass	1 oz. cooked weight	7
Shrimp	1 oz. cooked weight	6
Snapper	1 oz. cooked weight	8
Swordfish	1 oz. cooked weight	7 (2 fat)
Trout	1 oz. cooked weight	7 (2 fat)
Tuna steak	1 oz. cooked weight	8
Tuna in water, canned and drained	1 oz. cooked weight	7
Whitefish	1 oz. cooked weight	7 (2 fat)

CARBOHYDRATE SOURCES		
Food	Serving Size	Carbs
FRUIT/FRUIT JUICES		
Apple	½ medium	11
Apple juice	4 oz.	15
Apricots, dried	1 oz.	10
Apricots, fresh	3 medium	12
Banana	½ medium	14
Cantaloupe	1 cup	14
Cherries with pits	1 cup	13
Grapefruit	½ medium	11
Grapefruit juice	4 oz.	13
Grapes	1 cup	15
Kiwi	1 medium	12
Mango, peeled	2 oz.	10
Nectarine	1 medium	16
Orange	1 medium	17
Orange juice	4 oz.	14
Peach	1 medium	10
Pear	½ medium	13
Pineapple	½ cup	10
Pineapple juice	4 oz.	15
Plum	1 medium	9
Raisins	2 tbsp.	16
Strawberries	½ cup	6
Watermelon	1 cup	12
BREADS		
Bagel	1 large	43
Pita bread, white	1 slice	29
Pumpernickel bread	1 slice	16
Rye bread	1 slice	16
Wheat bread	1 slice	12

CARBOHYDRATE SOURCES, CONT'D.

Food	Serving Size	Carbs
CEREALS/GRAINS		
Cream of Wheat	1 cup	30
Grape-Nuts	1 oz.	24
Nutri-Grain	¾ cup	24
Oatmeal	½ cup dry weight	27
Puffed wheat	1 cup	11
Shredded Wheat	1 piece	19
PASTA/POTATOES/RICE		
Pasta, various types	1 oz. uncooked	21
Potato, baked	½ medium	26
Potato, boiled	1 medium, peeled	27
Potato, sweet	½ cup baked	25
Rice, brown	½ cup cooked	25
Rice, white	½ cup cooked	25
Rice, white (instant)	½ cup cooked	20
Rice cakes	1 regular	9
Yam	½ cup boiled or baked	19
VEGETABLES		
Asparagus	1 cup or 12 spears	9
Beans, green	½ cup raw, boiled, or canned	4
Beets, sliced	½ cup boiled	9
Broccoli	1 cup cooked	10
Brussels sprouts	1 cup cooked	13
Cabbage	1 cup cooked	7
Carrots	½ cup or 1 whole raw	8
Cauliflower	1 cup cooked or raw	6
Celery	1 cup or 4 stalks	4
Corn	¼ cup cooked	7
Cucumber	2 cups	6
Eggplant	1 cup cooked	6

CARBOHYDRATE SOURCES

Food	Serving Size	Carbs
VEGETABLES		
Lentils	¼ cup cooked or dry	10
Lettuce, iceberg	½ head	6
Lettuce, romaine	3 cups	4
Mushrooms (cooked)	1 cup	8
Mushrooms (raw)	1 cup	3
Onions	½ cup raw	6
Peas	½ cup cooked or dry	6
Peppers, green	1 pepper	4
Peppers, red	1 pepper	4
Radishes	4 medium	1
Sauerkraut	1 cup canned	10
Spinach	1 cup cooked	7
Tomatoes	1 raw	5
Squash, summer	1 cup cooked	8
Squash, winter	½ cup baked	9

FAT SOURCES		
Food	**Serving Size**	**Fat**
NUTS/NUT BUTTERS		
Almonds	½ oz.	8
Almond butter	½ oz.	8
Cashews	½ oz.	7
Cashew butter	½ oz.	7
Macadamia nuts	¼ oz.	6
Peanuts	½ oz.	7
Peanut butter	1 tbsp.	8
Walnuts	½ oz.	8
OILS		
Oil, almond	1 tsp.	5
Oil, canola	1 tsp.	5
Oil, corn	1 tsp.	5
Oil, olive	1 tsp.	5
Oil, peanut	1 tsp.	5
Oil, sesame	1 tsp.	5
OTHER		
Avocado	1 oz. trimmed	5
Guacamole	1 tbsp.	6
Olives	1 oz. green, pitted	4

ABOUT THE AUTHOR

To distill **Frank Sepe** in brief isn't as easy as one may think. Sure, as one of the most photographed physique models of all time, Frank has graced hundreds of fitness magazine covers (*Muscle and Fitness, MuscleMag International, Iron Man, Muscular Development,* and *American Health & Fitness,* to name a few), romance-book jackets, and fitness encyclopedias; and he's been the subject of some 500 fan Websites. But this isn't nearly the full picture . . . not by a long shot.

Frank was the resident fitness expert for ESPN2's *Cold Pizza.* He's also a highly respected writer who's the author of *The TRUTH: The Only Fitness Book You'll Ever Need* and *Frank Sepe's ABS-olutely Perfect Plan for a Flatter Stomach;* a contributing editor and monthly columnist for leading magazines *(MuscleMag International, American Health & Fitness);* the editor and fitness director for *Health Smart Today* and *Health Watchers* magazines, as well as publications for sports and training giant AXL (Athletic Extreme Living); and a consultant/fitness source for dozens of TV, news, and radio shows, as well as for the *Oxygen, Cosmopolitan,* and *American Curves* women's-fitness publications.

He's also a working actor *(The Devil and Daniel Webster, Carlito's Way)* who's made frequent TV guest appearances *(Live with Regis and Kelly, The Howard Stern Show, Late Night with Conan O'Brien, The Rick Sanchez Show).* He maintains private personal-training clients (including celebrities and professional athletes) and a full schedule as a spokesperson for fitness giant MET-Rx—all while promoting accredited physique programs. To contact Frank, please e-mail: **mail@franksepe.com** or go to **www.franksepe.com.**

Finally, please tune in to Frank's weekly program on **HayHouseRadio.com®.**

NOTES

NOTES

NOTES

NOTES

NOTES

NOTES

NOTES

NOTES

NOTES

NOTES

We hope you enjoyed this Hay House book. If you'd like to receive a free catalog featuring additional Hay House books and products, or if you'd like information about the Hay Foundation, please contact:

Hay House, Inc.
P.O. Box 5100
Carlsbad, CA 92018-5100

(760) 431-7695 or **(800) 654-5126**
(760) 431-6948 (fax) or **(800) 650-5115 (fax)**
www.hayhouse.com® • **www.hayfoundation.org**

Published and distributed in Australia by: Hay House Australia Pty. Ltd. • 18/36 Ralph St. • Alexandria NSW 2015 • *Phone:* 612-9669-4299 • *Fax:* 612-9669-4144 • www.hayhouse.com.au

Published and distributed in the United Kingdom by: Hay House UK, Ltd. • Unit 62, Canalot Studios • 292 Kensal Rd., London W10 5BE • *Phone:* 44-20-8962-1230 • *Fax:* 44-20-8962-1239 • www.hayhouse.co.uk

Published and distributed in the Republic of South Africa by: Hay House SA (Pty), Ltd., P.O. Box 990, Witkoppen 2068 • *Phone/Fax:* 27-11-706-6612 • orders@psdprom.co.za

Published in India by: Hay House Publications (India) Pvt. Ltd., 3 Hampton Court, A-Wing, 123 Wodehouse Rd., Colaba, Mumbai 400005 • *Phone:* 91 (22) 22150557 or 22180533 • *Fax:* 91 (22) 22839619 • www.hayhouseindia.co.in

Distributed in India by: Media Star, 7 Vaswani Mansion, 120 Dinshaw Vachha Rd., Churchgate, Mumbai 400020 • *Phone:* 91 (22) 22815538-39-40 • *Fax:* 91 (22) 22839619 • booksdivision@mediastar.co.in

Distributed in Canada by: Raincoast • 9050 Shaughnessy St., Vancouver, B.C. V6P 6E5 • *Phone:* (604) 323-7100 • *Fax:* (604) 323-2600 • www.raincoast.com

Tune in to **HayHouseRadio.com®** for the best in inspirational talk radio featuring top Hay House authors! And, sign up via the Hay House USA Website to receive the Hay House online newsletter and stay informed about what's going on with your favorite authors. You'll receive bimonthly announcements about: Discounts and Offers, Special Events, Product Highlights, Free Excerpts, Giveaways, and more!
www.hayhouse.com®